AIDS: A Guide for the Primary Physician

Edited by **King K. Holmes**, M
and **Arno G. Motulsky**, M.D.,

AIDS: A Guide for the Primary Physician

University of Washington Press   Seattle and London

AIDS: A Guide for the Primary Physician was originally published as Volume 13, Number 1 (Winter 1987) of *University of Washington Medicine,* published biannually by the University of Washington School of Medicine, Seattle, Washington 98195. Editor: Arno G. Motulsky, M.D., Sc.D; Editorial Board: Herbert Abelson, M.D., Richard Anderson, M.D., Alexander Clowes, M.D., Wayne Crill, M.D., Raymond Fink, M.D., Jan Hirschmann, M.D., Thomas Inui, M.D., John Sherris, M.D.; Managing Editor: Sabrina Porter Lindquist; Design: Pat Hansen Design

Photographs provided by:
All of You photographic services (pp. 11, 43)
UW Department of Medical History and Ethics (p. 48)
Mary Levin (pp. 55, 58)
Cynthia Taylor (p. 56)
Betty Udesen, *Seattle Times* (p. 14)
George White (p. 45)
World Health Organization (p. 62)

Contents

Preface

by King K. Holmes, M.D., Ph.D.

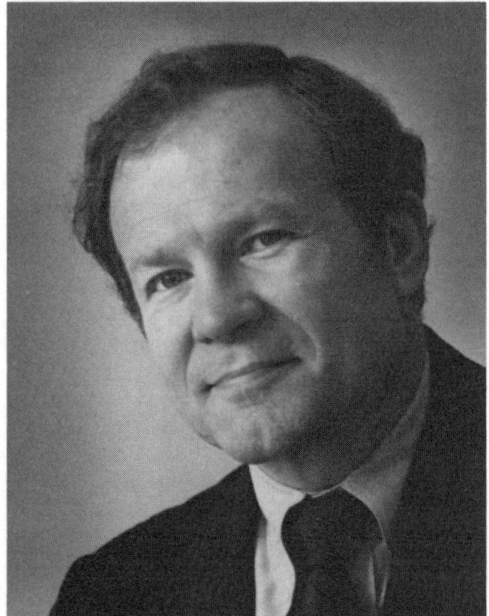

Which physicians should take care of patients with acquired immunodeficiency syndrome (AIDS)? Vaccines and curative antiviral therapy are not on the immediate horizon. Academic medical centers in some U.S. metropolitan areas are already overwhelmed by patients with AIDS. Special AIDS clinics are swamped and cannot alone cope with the growing number of cases.

More and more AIDS clinics are popping up in hospitals around the country. Some are directed by infectious disease specialists, but many are directed by general medicine internists or others involved in primary care medicine. Infectious disease specialists are skilled in managing opportunistic infections and are learning about the use of new antiviral drugs for human immunodeficiency virus (HIV) infections. However, they have no unique qualifications in management of opportunistic neoplasms or neuropsychiatric disorders, in delivery of long-term primary care, or in case management of complex social needs. Furthermore, infectious disease specialists are vastly outnumbered by the rapidly expanding numbers of persons with HIV infections. Thus, the growing consensus is that primary care physicians, including both generalists and specialists, will play a central role in managing HIV infections. Primary physicians are experienced in coordinating subspecialty consultations for multisystem diseases and in managing the complex, long-term psychosocial needs of patients with progressive, fatal illness.

To effectively manage technical aspects of treating AIDS, physicians will need ready access to new information on diagnosis, treatment, and case management issues. This volume is the first effort in a new, ongoing AIDS training program for health care workers in the Northwest. A recent grant from the Health Resources and Services Administration will enable an AIDS Educational Training Program to be established at the University of Washington School of Medicine and the Oregon Health Sciences University School of Medicine for training clinicians in Washington, Oregon, Alaska, Montana and Idaho. Similar regional training programs have been established at the schools of medicine of the University of California at Davis, New York University, and Ohio State University. As discussed in this volume by Drs. Koop, Matheny and Hostetter, the new regional programs will train primary care practitioners and allied health personnel in the medical, psychiatric and psychosocial aspects of AIDS and related conditions, thereby increasing the number of primary providers who are willing and able to manage and counsel AIDS patients.

The valued support of SAFECO Insurance Companies, the WAMI Area Health Education Center Program, the University of Washington School of Social Work, and the King County Medical Society has enabled us to considerably expand the scope of this volume. It includes a variety of basic science, clinical, public health, and social and ethical issues as a foundation for further knowledge in this rapidly evolving field. While not exhaustively comprehensive, the material is oriented toward the practicing clinician. Even the articles dealing with basic science—those on retroviruses, laboratory diagnosis, and antiviral chemotherapy—present concise reviews of new material that is fast becoming essential for the clinician who wants to know more than the patient. Terms such as "p24 antigen," "reverse transcriptase inhibitors" and "CD4 count" will soon be as familiar to us all as calcium channel blockers and antinuclear antibodies. This volume includes useful clinical guidelines and identifies some of the local experts who are available to give further help. We hope you will refer to it often and will contact a local source when you need more information.

Dr. Holmes is chief of Harborview Medical Center's Department of Medicine and professor and vice-chairman of the University of Washington Department of Medicine.

Epidemiology of Acquired Immunodeficiency Syndrome and Human Immunodeficiency Virus Infection in the United States and the Pacific Northwest

by H. Hunter Handsfield, M.D.

Before the cause of acquired immunodeficiency syndrome (AIDS) was identified and with incomplete knowledge of the full spectrum of human immunodeficiency virus (HIV) infection, a definition of AIDS was developed by the Centers for Disease Control for the purpose of epidemiologic surveillance. In essence, AIDS was defined by the occurrence of certain serious, systemic infections or malignancies that predict a defect in cell-mediated immunity in a person without known cause for immune deficiency. Despite subsequent modifications, this definition has proved effective for epidemiologic purposes. However, it was originally assumed and subsequently confirmed that overt AIDS, according to this definition, encompasses only a minority of all HIV infections.

AIDS and HIV infection in the United States and the Pacific Northwest

As of October 1987, the AIDS cases that met the epidemiologic definition numbered more than 42,000 in the United States, and almost 25,000 of those persons (59 percent) had died. The rate of new AIDS cases reported to the Centers for Disease Control (CDC) accelerated through 1984, followed by a continued but less sharp increase through late 1987. The CDC AIDS surveillance case definition was revised in August 1987 to encompass presumptively diagnosed opportunistic infections and a larger proportion of Group IV HIV infections (see "Clinical Manifestations and Approach to Management of HIV Infection and AIDS," Table I, page 27). This revision will shift the number of reported cases upward both nationally and regionally.

Based on cases reported through June 1986, the CDC projected a total of 270,000 cases through 1991, with 179,000 cumulative deaths. In the Pacific Northwest, we can expect a cumulative total of about 7,000 cases with approximately 4,000 deaths by the end of 1991. Because there is usually a lapse of several years between acquisition of HIV and the development of overt AIDS, most of these cases will occur in persons who are already infected. Thus, complete curtailment of HIV transmission now would have only a minor effect on the number of AIDS cases in the next five years. The 1991 projections also ignore AIDS-related complex (ARC) and other clinical syndromes that re-

quire medical care; such cases substantially outnumber those of overt AIDS.

AIDS cases have been reported in all U.S. states and territories but are not uniformly distributed. Although the majority of cases have occurred in a few cities (Table I), increasing numbers are being reported in other areas, including suburban and rural settings. The most rapidly rising incidence currently is in these other areas, a trend that will continue.

The occurrence of AIDS in the Pacific Northwest has paralleled that in the country as a whole. For example, Figure 1 shows the reported cases and deaths in Washington state from the first cases in 1982 through the first nine months of 1987. The accelerating case rate in Washington is similar to that occurring nationally and throughout the Pacific Northwest. Table II summarizes the reported cases and projections through 1991 for the five Pacific Northwest states. (The 95-percent confidence intervals around these projections are very broad and these figures should be considered only very rough estimates.) Of the 791 regional cases, 565 (71 percent) were reported in the Seattle and Portland metropolitan areas (King and Multnomah counties). As in the rest of the country, however, the most rapid growth is occurring in smaller cities and in rural areas. The number of Pacific Northwest cases outside the Seattle and Portland areas has increased eight-fold since 1984, compared with a five-fold rise in King and Multnomah counties.

Risk groups

Table III shows the risk-group categorization of adults with AIDS both nationally and in King County, Wash. Throughout the United States and most industrialized countries, homosexual and bisexual men account for the majority of AIDS cases. Heterosexual intravenous (IV) drug abusers are the second largest group, fol-

Table I Reported AIDS Cases by Standard Metropolitan Statistical Area (SMSA) of Residence*, through August 31, 1987

			Reported Cases	
Rank	SMSA	Cases per 100,000 Population	1987	Cumulative Total
1	San Francisco	123	719	4,007
2	New York	118	1,569	10,751
3	Jersey City, NJ	83	82	462
4	Miami	70	155	1,149
5	Fort Lauderdale, FL	52	123	529
6	Newark, NJ	49	174	957
7	Los Angeles	47	678	3,551
8	Houston	46	236	1,346
9	Washington, D.C.	40	290	1,217
10	Atlanta	33	147	666
11	New Orleans	30	75	354
12	San Diego	28	136	526
13	Dallas	27	222	796
14	Seattle	25	105 +	403 +
15	Boston	23	147	637
16	Denver	22	87	353
17	Nassau-Suffolk, NY	20	98	515
18	Anaheim, CA	18	86	338
19	Philadelphia	17	156	794
20	Chicago	14	223	991
21	Remainder of U.S.	7	2,383	11,024

*Ranked according to cases per 100,000 population (1980 census)

+Differences with Seattle-King County Department of Public Health figures reflect delays in reporting or data tabulation.

Dr. Handsfield directs the Sexually Transmitted Disease Control Program of the Seattle-King County Department of Public Health and is an associate professor of medicine and an adjunct associate professor of epidemiology at the University of Washington.

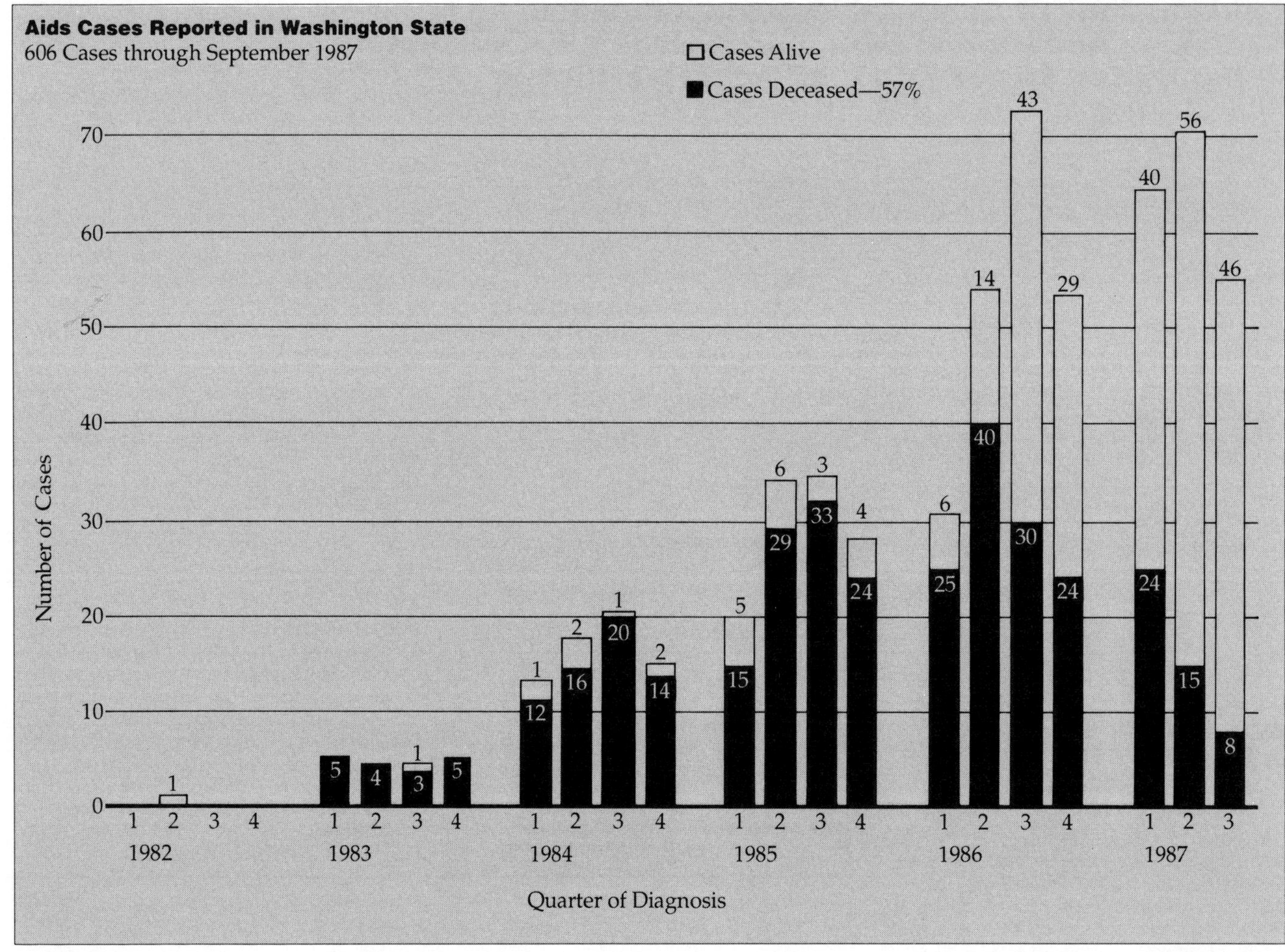

FIGURE 1.

lowed by homosexual male IV drug abusers. In the United States, IV drug abuse is a common independent risk factor in several Eastern metropolitan areas, but not in the Northwest (see Table III). Most IV drug abusers probably are less mobile than most homosexual men, resulting in slower spread of HIV from IV drug abusers in the East to those in the West. It is also possible that there is less sharing of injection equipment in the West. However, increased numbers of heterosexual IV drug abusers with AIDS or HIV infection have been documented recently in several cities in the western United States, including Seattle and Portland.

Hemophiliacs constitute only 1 percent of AIDS cases. Nationally, however, there are only about 14,000 hemophiliacs who require regular treatment with blood products; among these, more than 2 percent have acquired AIDS and at least 60 percent are infected with HIV. Thus, on a population basis, hemophiliacs may be the group at highest risk. Pasteurization of clotting factor concentrates, increased use of cryoprecipitate, and serological screening of blood donors have now eliminated the risk of HIV exposure for hemophiliacs who have not yet been infected with HIV.

Persons who received blood transfusions between 1978 and mid-1985 account for about 2 percent of the cases nationally. In contrast to the small number of hemophiliacs, however, more than 25 million persons received blood transfusions during that time, so the actual risk among transfusion recipients was very low. Current blood-banking methods, including voluntary self-exclusion of persons at risk for AIDS and universal testing of donors for HIV infection, are almost 100-percent reliable in excluding infected donors. Unfortunately, the pool of persons infected by blood and blood products prior to 1985 will continue to generate cases of AIDS for many years.

Approximately 4 percent of AIDS cases nationally and less than 1 percent locally are attributed to heterosexual acquisition of HIV. These proportions may be inflated by persons who deny high-risk behavior or do not realize they belong to other risk groups. For example, most of the males in this category are Haitian natives who probably were infected with HIV before they immigrated; their situation may not reflect transmission risks in the United States. Most women with sexually acquired AIDS have been sexual partners of infected IV drug abusers. Although there is clear evidence of bidirectional heterosexual transmission of HIV, it is likely that the virus is more readily transmitted sexually from men to women than the reverse. The extent of the problem of sustained heterosexual transmission of HIV in the United States is not yet known. In Washington state, only two cases to date have been attributed to heterosexual acquisition.

The occurrence of AIDS in persons with no identified risk factor is often cited as evidence for HIV transmission by contact that does not involve the exchange of blood or sexual secretions. However, studies by the CDC and others have shown that the majority of these patients belonged to, but nonetheless denied connection with, established risk groups. Because the most common risk factors are viewed negatively by much of society, it would be surprising if such denial did not occur frequently. In other cases, patients were unaware of known risk factors, as might occur when a woman has had a sexual relationship with a man who, unknown to her, was bisexual or used IV drugs.

Among the 595 cases of AIDS in children reported in the United States, 73 percent had a parent at risk; most of these were infected *in utero* or during delivery. Fourteen percent of the children with AIDS acquired it by transfusion; 9 percent were hemophiliacs; and the remaining 4 percent had no identified risk. One case of early childhood HIV infection has been attributed to transmission from an infected mother through nursing. Only four cases of AIDS have been confirmed in children under 13 years old in the five Pacific Northwest states; all were born to infected mothers.

As suggested by the characteristics of the groups at risk of AIDS, the overwhelming majority of cases occur in males, who account for 93 percent of adult cases nationally and 97 percent of cases in the Pacific Northwest. Both nationally and locally, approximately 88 percent of AIDS patients are 20 to 49 years old; nearly half of all cases are between the ages of 30 and 39. Nationally, 61 percent are white, 24 percent are black, and 14 percent are Hispanic. However, the incidence of AIDS and the prevalence of HIV infection are substantially higher in blacks and Hispanics than in whites, largely due to the ethnic characteristics of IV drug abusers. In the Pacific Northwest, more than 90 percent of AIDS patients are white, and 2 to 4 percent each are black, Hispanic, or members of other ethnic groups.

Prevalence of HIV infection

Numerous studies have assessed the prevalence of HIV infection in various populations without overt AIDS. Interpretation of nearly all these surveys has been hampered because the persons studied were not representative of the population as a whole. For example, most studies of homosexual and bisexual men have involved volunteers for research studies or people who sought HIV serological testing for personal reasons. Data from blood donors exclude persons who admit they belong to AIDS risk groups.

Nonetheless, these studies have contributed to an understanding of the broad outlines of HIV infection and risk. The prevalence of HIV infection in homosexual and bisexual men studied in most urban areas of the United States varies from 15 to 70 percent. Among gay men seeking testing and counseling at the AIDS Prevention Project of the Seattle-King County Department of Public Health, test results for 123 (23 percent) of 534 men were positive for HIV antibody. By contrast, HIV infection has been documented in 45 to 55 percent of gay men tested who attended the Seattle-King County Sexually Transmitted Diseases (STD) Clinic at Harborview Medical Center or the Seattle Gay Clinic. The AIDS Prevention Project group is more likely to have been at relatively low risk, whereas the STD Clinic and Seattle Gay Clinic serve persons at relatively high risk. Therefore, the true prevalence of HIV infection in Seattle-King County gay men probably is between these extremes, most likely between 25 and 35 percent.

The proportion of HIV seropositives has been stable for two years at the AIDS Prevention Project and for more than four years at the STD Clinic. Thus, the frequency of new HIV infections apparently is substantially lower now than it was before risk-reduction messages were widely publicized. In San Francisco, more than 10 percent of gay men probably became infected with HIV each year from 1980 to 1984; more recent studies suggest that the current risk approximates 1 percent annually. A similar change probably has occurred in the Pacific Northwest.

The few studies of IV drug abusers suggest prevalences of HIV infection of 50 percent or more in the East Coast cities with the most drug-related AIDS cases. Prevalences are substantially lower in Midwestern and Western cities, but recently appear to be growing. Among 95 heterosexual IV drug abusers tested at the Seattle-King County AIDS Prevention Project in 1986 and 1987, four (4 percent) were seropositive. Nationally, the prevalence of HIV infection in hemophiliacs is about 80 percent among those who were treated with pooled factor VIII concentrate. Fortunately, the prevalence is substantially lower among hemophiliacs in the Seattle area, because for several years the Puget Sound Blood Center has used cryoprecipitated factor VIII, which had a lower risk of HIV contamination than concentrate.

Only a few studies have examined populations whose only apparent risk was heterosexual exposure. All of these showed low prevalences of HIV infection. For example, among 343 women and heterosexual men who visited the Seattle-King County/Harborview STD Clinic in November and December 1986 and 307 who visited in August and September 1987, none had positive results in HIV tests. In Brooklyn, N.Y., an STD clinic that serves a large population of HIV-infected, heterosexual IV drug abusers found no HIV infection among more than 100 male patients who did not use IV drugs. The low rates of infection in these populations, selected on the basis of having or being exposed to sexually transmitted infections, suggest that heterosexual transmission of HIV is not yet common in the United States.

Among 789,578 military recruits throughout the country tested from October 1985 through December 1986, 1,186 (0.15 percent) were positive. The rate of positivity dropped slightly during the latter part of this period, especially among white men. There is great geographic variation in the prevalence of HIV infection in recruits; the highest rates occur in metropolitan areas with the greatest numbers of overt AIDS cases. Although military personnel and recruits deny illicit drug use and homosexuality, many of these infected persons nevertheless belong to recognized risk groups. However, an unknown proportion may have been infected through heterosexual activity. It is not known whether the recent small drop in the rate of infected recruits is due to stabilization of the risk of HIV infection or because the number of homosexual men and IV drug abusers who apply for military service has dropped.

The prevalence of HIV infection in volunteer (non-paid) blood donors is extremely low. In blood donation programs administered nationally by the American Red Cross, the prevalence of HIV infection in prospective donors is approximately 0.025 percent. Among 211,000 potential donors at all five Washington state blood blanks in 1986, there were 24 confirmed seropositives (0.011 percent), and similar figures have been documented elsewhere in the Pacific Northwest. However, these figures under-

Table II Reported and Projected AIDS Cases in the Pacific Northwest

State	Reported Cases*	Projected Cases through 1991†
Washington	516	5000
Oregon	213	1400
Alaska	43	—
Idaho	11	—
Montana	8	—
Total	791	7000

*Through September 8, 1987; figures do not reflect the 1987 expansion of the Centers for Disease Control (CDC) AIDS surveillance case definition.

†Based on the percentage of nationally reported cases from each state and the CDC projection of nationally reported cases through 1991 (Morgan, M. 1986. AIDS: current and future trends. *Pub Health Rep* 101:459-65). Adjusted for the expanded CDC AIDS surveillance case definition and for an estimated 20-percent underreporting of cases. Case numbers to date for Alaska, Idaho and Montana are too small for accurate state-by-state projections.

Table III AIDS Risk Groups

Group	Percent of Reported Cases of AIDS	
	United States	Seattle-King Co.
Homosexual/bisexual male	63.9	87.5
Intravenous drug abuser	15.0	0.6
Homosexual male/intravenous drug abuser	7.1	8.5
Hemophilia	0.9	0.6
Heterosexual cases	3.9	0.6
Transfusion/blood product exposure	2.0	0.9
Undetermined	3.2	1.2

estimate the overall prevalence of HIV infection in society, because members of recognized risk groups are asked not to donate blood. Nonetheless, almost all voluntary donors with HIV infection, both locally and nationally, have had traditional risk factors that were denied or unrecognized.

It is currently estimated that about one in 500,000 units of blood collected in the United States is contaminated with HIV but is falsely seronegative. In some cases, this has been shown to involve recently infected donors who had not yet seroconverted. It is likely that the prevalence of seronegative contaminated blood is somewhat higher in areas with high incidences of AIDS (for example, New York City) and even less than one in 500,000 in the Pacific Northwest and other areas where HIV infection is relatively uncommon.

The CDC estimates that between 1 million and 2 million people in the United States currently are infected with HIV. It is likely that the incidence of new infections is growing less rapidly than it did from 1978 to 1985, due to widespread behavioral changes among homosexual men. However, even if HIV transmission to new individuals were immediately halted, it is likely—barring development of therapy able to alter the progression of HIV infection—that at least 500,000 and perhaps 1 million or more of those Americans who are already infected will develop overt AIDS in the next several years.

Transmission of HIV

The modes of transmission of HIV, summarized in Table IV, may be surmised in general terms from knowledge of risk groups. Receptive anal intercourse carries the highest risk of HIV acquisition for homosexual men. For women, both vaginal and anal intercourse are risky, but anal in-

Table IV Modes of Transmission of Human Immunodeficiency Virus

---

1. Sexual contact
   —Intercourse (vaginal, anal)
   —Oral-genital practices
   —Kissing ?

---

2. Blood-borne transmission
   —Transfusion, blood products
   —Intravenous drug abuse with needle-sharing
   —Accidental injury (health care personnel)
   —Cutaneous contact (rare; probably requires unrecognized wound or mucous membrane exposure)

---

3. *In-utero* and perinatal transmission

---

4. Artificial insemination

---

5. Organ transplantation

---

6. Nursing (via breast milk)

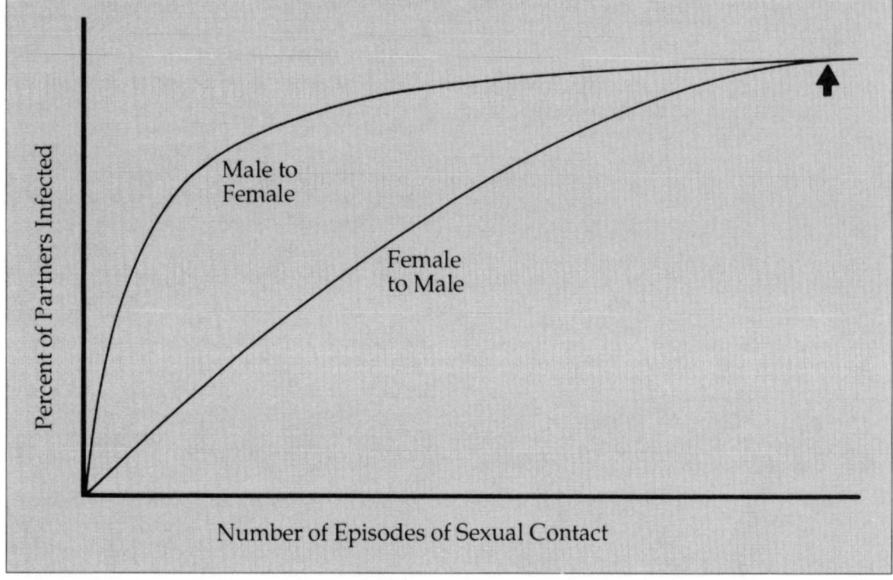

FIGURE 2. Hypothetical patterns of HIV transmission.

tercourse may be more so. The insertive male partner may have a somewhat lower risk of acquiring HIV from an infected person, but the epidemic of HIV infection in heterosexual men in equatorial Africa and the occurrence of HIV infection in some male sex partners of infected women in North America leave no doubt that the insertive partner can be infected. One study indicates a risk for the receptive (oral) partner in fellatio with an infected person, especially if intra-oral ejaculation occurs. Kissing and other forms of sexual expression have not been definitively documented to be risky. However, most people participate in several sexual practices, and the risk for anal or vaginal intercourse may statistically overwhelm those of other activities.

Accordingly, it is believed that any sexual contact that allows infected secretions or blood to be deposited into any body cavity, under the skin, or into the bloodstream carries a risk of virus transmission. HIV is present in high concentrations in the semen and blood of infected persons, and in somewhat lower concentrations in female cervical secretions. It is present infrequently and in much lower concentrations in urine, saliva, tears and breast milk.

The potential for sustained heterosexual transmission of HIV in the United States and western Europe is intensely debated among epidemiologists studying AIDS. Bidirectional heterosexual HIV transmission is common in equatorial Africa, where it accounts for the majority of all AIDS cases (see "A Global Perspective on AIDS" on page 60). On the other hand, very few heterosexually acquired AIDS cases have been reported so far in American men; most cases attributed to heterosexual acquisition have occurred in the female partners of IV drug abusers or bisexual men. As for most sexually transmitted infections, it is likely that HIV is more efficiently transmitted from men to women than vice versa, probably because infected semen is deposited directly into the vagina.

Figure 2 compares hypothetical patterns of HIV transmission from male to female and the reverse. Data exist to support this pattern for gonorrhea, and I believe it likely that it holds for *Chlamydia trachomatis* and other pathogens transmitted via semen and cervical secretions. The prevalence of infection in men and women in stable relationships—that is, beyond the point designated by the arrow—may ultimately be similar despite the greater efficiency of transmission from men to women than the reverse. But in casual sexual relationships, the setting responsible for most sexually transmitted diseases, women are at substantially greater risk than men. Thus, studies documenting that steady male partners of infected women have HIV infection prevalences similar to those in steady female partners of infected men do not necessarily indicate similar efficiencies of HIV transmission. If this pattern applies to HIV, person-to-person transmission of the virus will be less well-sustained in heterosexual men and women than in homosexual men or IV drug abusers.

Various cofactors for HIV transmission may exist in Africa and in homosexual men that are absent in American heterosexuals, and help to reconcile differences in the epidemiology of HIV infection. For example, ulcerative disease of the genitals or the anal area—due primarily to herpes and syphilis in Europe and the United States, and to chancroid and syphilis in Africa—appear to enhance the efficiency of bidirectional HIV transmission (see "A Global Perspective on AIDS" on page 60). These conditions probably are substantially more common in homosexual men and in some African men and women than in most Western heterosexual populations. Other unrecognized biological or behavioral cofactors also may contribute to differences in the rate of sexual transmission of HIV.

Despite publicity about three health care workers who acquired HIV infection without an obvious route of entry into their bloodstreams, this phenomenon appears to be an uncommon exception, and these persons failed to follow standard infection control practices to reduce the occupational risk of infection. The risk of acquiring HIV infection by contaminated needle-stick injury is less than 1 percent (see "Infection Control in AIDS" on page 55). These cases confirm the need to handle contaminated sharp instruments with care and to wear rubber gloves when handling secretions or blood. Masks, goggles and other protective clothing also are indicated if there is a risk that infected materials may be splattered or dispersed.

There is strong epidemiologic evidence that HIV is not transmitted with detectable frequency by non-intimate contact with infected persons. One study involved 101 members of households of persons with AIDS or other forms of HIV infection. None were sex partners or shared drug injection equipment with the infected persons. The duration of contact with the infected persons ranged from three months to four years, with a median of 22 months. The only infected household member was a young child whose mother had AIDS and who was believed to have acquired HIV at birth. Among the 100 uninfected household members, more than 90 percent shared kitchen or toilet facilities with the infected person, 80 percent regularly hugged or kissed the infected person, about half shared drinking or eating utensils, and many assisted in terminal care of the AIDS patient. Seven percent shared toothbrushes and 9 percent shared razors with the AIDS patient. If these forms of contact over an average of nearly two years resulted in no HIV transmission, it is clear that common, daily contact with an HIV carrier—for example, among co-workers or school classmates—carries a negligible risk of infection. Similar results have been reported among household contacts in central Africa and in a French boarding school that housed a hemophiliac boy with HIV infection. Although some people fear that mosquitoes or other blood-feeding arthropods might transmit HIV, no such transmission has been detected in studies of household contacts in areas where mosquitoes are prevalent, such as in equatorial Africa and southern Florida.

Summary

Sexual transmission accounts for the largest group of reported AIDS cases. The second largest group is comprised of persons exposed to blood or to therapeutic products derived from blood. Transmission thus requires direct placement of infected material into the bloodstream, under the skin, or into a body orifice. It probably accounts for AIDS in newborns from their infected mothers; in IV drug abusers who share injection equipment; and in transfusion recipients, hemophiliacs, recipients of transplanted organs, and nosocomially infected health professionals following injury with a sharp instrument.

Additional Reading

Wood, R.W. and Collier, A.C. 1987. Acquired immunodeficiency syndrome. Chapter 5 in Handsfield, H.H. (ed); Sexually Transmitted Diseases. *Infectious Disease Clinics of North America*, Vol. 1. Saunders, Philadelphia.

Centers for Disease Control. 1986. Update: Acquired immunodeficiency syndrome—United States. *Morbid Mortal Weekly Rep* 35:757.

Friedland, G.H., Saltzman, B.R., Rogers, M.F. *et al.* 1986. Lack of transmission of HTLV-III/LAV infection to household contacts of patients with AIDS or AIDS-related complex with oral candidiasis. *N Engl J Med* 314:344.

Quinn, T.C., Piot, P., McCormick, J.B. *et al.* 1987. Serologic and immunologic studies in patients with AIDS in North America and Africa. *JAMA* 257:2617-2621.

Institute of Medicine, National Academy of Sciences. 1986. Confronting AIDS: Directions for Public Health, Health Care, and Research. National Academy Press, Washington, D.C.

Kreiss, J.K., Koech, D., Plummer, F.A. *et al.* 1986. AIDS virus infection in Nairobi prostitutes. *N Engl J Med* 314:414.

U.S. Public Health Service. 1986. The Coolfont Report: A PHS plan for the prevention and control of AIDS and the AIDS virus. *Pub Health Rep* 101:342.

The Public Health Response to AIDS

by Robert W. Wood, M.D.

Public health officials and primary physicians can take steps on three levels to control acquired immunodeficiency syndrome (AIDS). These levels include controlling disease transmission (primary prevention); controlling or delaying disease progression (secondary prevention); and controlling disease complications, including their impacts on the community (tertiary prevention).

At the first level, prevention of infection with human immunodeficiency virus (HIV) consists mainly of education about risk-taking behaviors. No drugs presently are capable of eradicating HIV infection, and the role of zidovudine (formerly known as azidothymidine or AZT) and other antiviral agents in preventing subsequent development of full-blown AIDS remains to be determined. Secondary prevention still is possible, however. Infected persons can be counseled to change behaviors that may activate HIV-infected lymphocytes, which may enhance HIV replication. Such behaviors include intravenous (IV) drug abuse and further exposure to sexually transmitted diseases through unprotected sex with multiple partners. Regular visits to primary care providers can facilitate early treatment of common infections. Tertiary prevention is possible mostly in a social context by developing efficient and comprehensive care systems to minimize the negative impacts of AIDS on the individual and on the population (Table I).

As this epidemic continues, it is clear that the resources of public health departments will not be fully sufficient to meet these needs. The proactive assistance of Northwest physicians in AIDS control is crucial if we are to succeed. This article is designed to help Northwest physicians fulfill their important role in AIDS control.

I will first describe the development of the Seattle-King County AIDS Project as a possible model for a public health response to AIDS. Other community responses to AIDS will then be discussed, followed by general approaches to AIDS prevention. Finally, I describe in more detail the AIDS Project's current resources and specific programs as a model for other Northwest cities.

Community response to AIDS

Seattle's first two cases of AIDS were identified in 1982. In 1983, the Seattle metropolitan area was one of the first in the nation to receive city and county council funds to establish an AIDS project (Table II). The

Dr. Wood is medical director of the AIDS Project and is a University of Washington associate professor of medicine and an adjunct associate professor of health services. He is a member of Washington Gov. Booth Gardner's AIDS Task Force.

Table I AIDS Control Programs in Seattle/King County

Primary Prevention:

Education

    At-risk populations:

    —Risk reduction via media

    —One-to-one counseling

    —HIV antibody testing

    —Partner notification

    —Extended counseling

    —Information about services

    General community:

    —Diminish fear

    —Risk reduction

Secondary Prevention:

One-to-one counseling

Clinical services to seropositives

Experimental antiviral chemotherapy

Tertiary Prevention:

Mayor's AIDS Task Force

Comprehensive home support

Case management

Fear reduction

Seattle-King County Department of Public Health used the initial funds to open an AIDS telephone hotline, provide public presentations, develop information brochures, and establish an AIDS Assessment Clinic. The clinic was staffed by a nurse practitioner who interviewed, examined and advised concerned persons individually. Bus posters dealt with fear, the "secondary epidemic," by reassuring the community that "You Can't Get It By Casual Contact." The department also established the AIDS Advisory Task Force with representatives from local organizations of at-risk persons, primarily gay men. The task force works to improve information exchange among affected groups and to review AIDS programs and policies for community acceptance.

As AIDS antibody testing became routine in blood banks in 1985, the department set up alternative test sites where concerned persons could find out whether they had been infected with HIV. We added this service to the AIDS Assessment Clinic and contracted with existing gay health organizations locally to provide an additional test site. Local government hired a medical director for the AIDS Project.

The Department of Public Health also was awarded support from the Centers for Disease Control (CDC) to establish one of four

(now six) disease control demonstration projects. Cooperative agreements linked this early federal support to research demonstrating the impact and cost of various AIDS control strategies. The research is evaluating innovative risk-reduction ideas through program documentation and by measuring changes in knowledge, behavior, attitudes and HIV seroprevalence. In 1985, the department also obtained additional CDC funds to establish an active AIDS surveillance program with a project epidemiologist and support staff.

We began longitudinal cohort studies in 1986 to measure the changes in knowledge, behaviors and seroprevalence associated with AIDS control activities. In the process, we learned of the gay community's serious concerns about the potential for government list-keeping in such studies and in HIV antibody testing. Fearing that such concerns would limit participation, we negotiated to provide clinical services, antibody testing and research study participation anonymously as well as confidentially. Three-quarters of our current clients choose to be anonymously registered.

In 1986, the Robert Wood Johnson Foundation made $17.2 million available to nine metropolitan areas to develop comprehensive care programs for persons with AIDS and AIDS-related diseases. We were awarded a $1.4-million grant over four years beginning in 1987. Thus, by the beginning of this year, the AIDS Project had grown from $40,000 of initial city/county funds and two full-time staff to an annual budget of approximately $1.5 million and 16 full-time staff (Table II).

University of Washington efforts

The AIDS Project works in close cooperation with other community organizations and groups. The University of Washington (UW), with established expertise in infectious diseases and particularly in sexually transmitted diseases, took a major step into AIDS care by establishing an AIDS outpatient clinic at Seattle's Harborview Medical Center in 1985 and hiring a full-time social worker for AIDS case management. Clinic doctors also offered their AIDS expertise to Northwest physicians through MEDCON, a UW service for physicians in need of telephone consultation in specialized areas of medicine. The UW vice president for health sciences established an AIDS Advisory Committee in 1987 to coordinate the university's response to the AIDS epidemic.

Two examples illustrate the scope and diversity of the many AIDS research projects under way at the UW. In 1986, the UW established an AIDS Treatment Evaluation

Unit under the direction of Dr. Lawrence Corey, UW professor of laboratory medicine, microbiology and medicine. The unit was set up with funds from the National Institutes of Health and in cooperation with a city-wide consortium of physicians who care for persons with AIDS (see "Prospects in Anti-Retroviral Chemotherapy for Treatment of HIV Infection" on page 36). The National Institute of Mental Health awarded Dr. Lewayne Gilchrist, research associate professor in the UW School of Social Work, a grant in October 1986 to train Northwest health care providers in the psychosocial, neurologic and mental health aspects of HIV infection (see "Psychosocial Aspects of AIDS" on page 42). Other federal or private grants to UW faculty support research projects on neurologic and psychiatric manifestations of HIV infection, perinatal and heterosexual transmission of HIV infection in Africa, primate retrovirus infection models, the results of HIV screening by blood banks, and basic research on the retroviruses.

The role of volunteers and private foundations

Community volunteer organizations also have played an extremely important role in the development of King County AIDS programs. The gay community, the group most affected by AIDS, provided much of the early community structure, but many diverse groups have since become involved (Figure 1). The non-profit Northwest AIDS Foundation was created in 1983 and has grown from an annual budget of $35,000 to more than $500,000. It provides community AIDS education, financial and case-management support for persons with AIDS, and valuable advocacy for improved care systems.

Table II King County AIDS Programs

Funding Source:	(dollars in thousands)				
	1983	1984	1985	1986	1987
Seattle-King Co. Dept. of Public Health					
Seattle City Council	$16	$34	$76	$142	$153
King County Council	$25	$58	$114	$140	$139
Centers for Disease Control					
—Surveillance			$5	$70	$80
—Disease Prevention Demonstration Project			$5	$365	$720
Robert Wood Johnson Foundation Grant					$378
Total:	$41	$92	$200	$717	$1,470

There are many more. The Chicken Soup Brigade, a volunteer offshoot of the Seattle Gay Clinic, provides transportation and home support services for persons with AIDS. Seattle SHANTI, a local chapter of the San Francisco-based organization, provides personalized emotional support; the Seattle AIDS Support Group provides group support. Groups such as Parents & Friends of Lesbians and Gays, the Seattle Counseling Service, Volunteer Attorneys for People with AIDS, Shoulders, and the Open Worried-Well Group provide valuable support for persons with AIDS and those around them. The contributions from these volunteers, if financially quantified, likely could equal or exceed the government funds earmarked for AIDS.

General approaches to AIDS prevention

Primary prevention of communicable diseases is generally achieved through vaccines that prevent infection; drugs that eradicate the agent in carriers; and sanitary measures, vector elimination, disease screening, and education to prevent spread. Unfortunately, no vaccines or drugs are presently available to combat the spread of HIV. HIV is not spread by casual contact or insect vectors, so that sanitary measures or vector elimination are not important. Thus, screening and education are the cornerstones of HIV control presently.

Testing for HIV antibodies

The disease prevention value of screening for antibodies to HIV is controversial but anecdotally may be powerful. Most people develop measurable antibodies within two to 12 weeks of infection and will remain permanently infected and contagious.

Gays and others have expressed concern about testing for HIV antibodies. Without available treatment or vaccine, some people argue that serologic testing will serve only to subject persons who already are heavily stigmatized to further discrimination, including loss of insurance, housing or employment. Since experience has shown that testing can cause broken relationships, heightened anxiety or even suicide, they argue that *everyone*—especially those already at risk for infection—*should now be practicing only "safe sex."* (See "Psychosocial Aspects of AIDS," Table I, page 46, for "safe sex" guidelines.) If no one engaged in unprotected sex involving the exchange of body fluids with new partners, and if needle-sharing among IV drug abusers came to a halt, AIDS would not spread. Routine testing to prevent inadvertent spread of infection is not advocated even in health care settings, where *all persons should be assumed to be infected with potentially harmful organisms and should be handled similarly* (see "Infection Control in AIDS" on page 55). These arguments suggest that testing is seldom necessary except in situations where knowledge of HIV serostatus may be important to a patient's medical care.

On the other hand, many public health authorities have a strong sense that voluntary screening—combined with AIDS education—can be extremely helpful in motivating those at risk to adopt safer lifestyles. Some political officials have recently recommended routine or mandatory screening of certain groups. There is strong

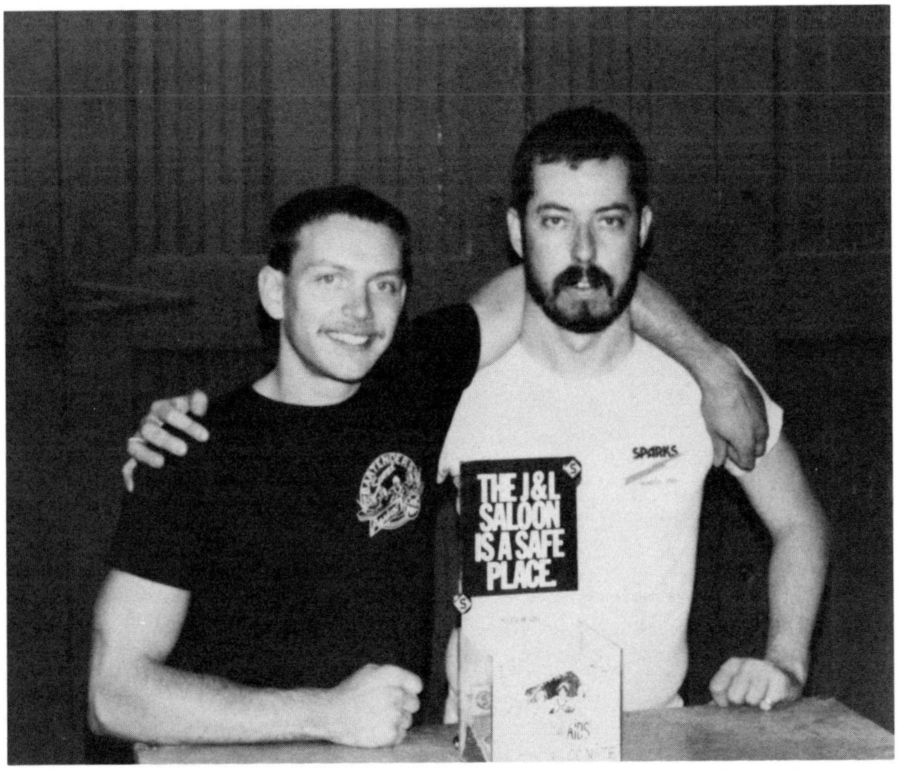

FIGURE 1. Seattle's "safe sex" education campaign is wide-ranging and includes these volunteers for "Bartenders Against AIDS."

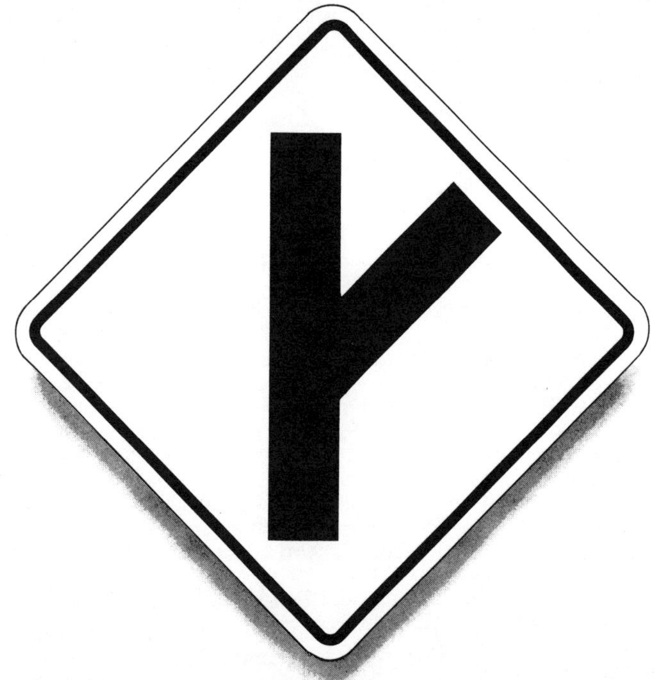

FIGURE 2. The Northwest AIDS Foundation and the AIDS Prevention Project target educational materials to gay as well as general audiences.

reason to believe that most mandatory screening—other than by blood banks—more likely will be counterproductive than useful in disease control. Persons most in need of counseling and AIDS screening are likely to be frightened away from programs offering such services by fears of governmental lists or rights infractions.

Testing and disease prevention

Several studies have explored the disease prevention value of testing. A study by Zones *et al* in San Francisco showed that persons with positive test results had more substantial intentions to practice safe sex than those with negative results or those who were not tested. Research in Baltimore by Fox, however, showed that persons who learned of a negative test result changed to safe sex more slowly than those who chose not to learn the result or who learned of a positive result. Thus, a positive test may promote safe sex but a negative test may provide false reassurance by suggesting invulnerability to HIV.

Because self-selection for testing may be strongly associated with intentions and testing effects—and because research on people must be ethical—the final answer to the question of testing's preventive value may be a long time coming. In the meantime, *testing should be done with the patient's understanding, at least verbal permission, and only with appropriate counseling.* Most public health and social scientists seem to believe that such one-to-one counseling, rather than the testing itself, produces screening's major disease-control effect. Persons reasonably likely to have positive test results should get substantial pre-test counseling that covers their histories, the pros and cons of testing, and their resources for dealing with a positive result. *Care providers should give test results in person to members of this high-risk group, never by phone or by mail.* Direct interaction permits more counseling and allows the caregiver to evaluate the patient's response.

To reduce disincentives for at-risk persons to use counseling and testing programs, the CDC has advocated federal leadership in a national effort to enact or change laws to protect the rights of the groups most affected by AIDS.

In association with the recent media emphasis on heterosexual spread of AIDS, we in Seattle have seen large numbers of frightened but very low-risk persons seeking HIV antibody testing. Programs designed for one-on-one counseling and testing of higher-risk persons have been overwhelmed by those whose test results are routinely negative and who simply could have been reassured and warned to "play it safe" from now on. Except to relieve media-generated anxiety, counseling and testing are rarely useful for persons outside high-risk groups, unless they have had sex with a person known to be antibody-positive. In fact, the vast majority of heterosexual transmission of AIDS is related to IV drug abuse on the East Coast. Although five (2 percent) of 229 women seen in the AIDS Assessment Clinic have been HIV-antibody-positive, all were in high-risk

groups: IV drug abusers, prostitutes, or sexual partners of persons known to be infected.

Education and counseling

Education is the major tool available for primary prevention of AIDS (Figure 2). Public health programs, with media assistance, have highlighted several important messages: that AIDS is preventable if people learn specifically how the disease is spread; that AIDS is not spread by casual contact such as occurs in public settings or in the workplace; and that compassionate and helpful approaches are essential as more and more people become afflicted.

The most specific messages are targeted to gay men and IV drug abusers, the groups at highest risk. However, U.S. Surgeon General C. Everett Koop—among others—has advocated that specific information be routinely provided to youth because many are sexually active before they leave high school (Figure 3). (A Harris poll recently indicated that 67 percent of teenagers are sexually active by age 17 and that only 47 percent of males and 25 percent of females report use of condoms.) Physicians could help considerably by providing AIDS information in their one-to-one patient contacts, especially with persons at risk for HIV infection. Such individualized attention, especially if consistent with public health messages, may have more profound impact than mass media approaches in reducing disease spread and fear while fostering care and compassion.

One-to-one counseling is especially important for high-risk populations. Physicians must first learn to recognize these individuals, who do not always fit common stereotypes. A study by the Kinsey Sex Research Institute showed that men who have sex with other men are a very diverse group that includes husbands, clergy, doctors and politicians. Similarly, IV drug abusers are not always easily recognizable. Care providers often must confront their own beliefs as they delve more deeply into their patients' lifestyles and sexual styles. To uncover HIV infection or risk, caregivers must be willing to discuss such issues and render appropriate assistance. Strong moralistic feelings impede data gathering and disease control.

Partner notification is used routinely to control such communicable diseases as gonorrhea and syphilis. For example, when a person with such a disease is identified, public health specialists ask the names of partners who may have been exposed and then notify them of the need to be evaluated and treated. Although no current treatment eradicates HIV, partner notification may still be useful when the persons exposed—especially women considering pregnancy and female partners of "closeted" bisexual men—are unaware of the risk.

We currently are developing policies and procedures that will facilitate such partner notification. Within the high-risk groups, however, such notification probably is not presently cost-effective and may politically sabotage our efforts to gain gay acceptance of counseling and voluntary testing. Since

public health recommendations have widely advertised that gay men and IV drug abusers seek individual counseling and evaluation, partner notification is unlikely to recommend anything new. Practitioners caring for members of high-risk communities should train each index case, whether seropositive or not, to recruit sexual or needle-sharing partners to spread the word about the need for all to undergo counseling and evaluation.

Some individuals who cannot easily change to low-risk behaviors may need extended counseling. Investigators are exploring how sexual behaviors can be considered and treated as addictions, as are cigarette smoking and alcohol abuse. Despite evidence of substantial changes in behaviors of gay men and IV drug abusers, some continue to take risks despite their knowledge of the possible consequences. (As of 1986, about 10 percent of gay men in San Francisco continued to engage in unprotected passive anal intercourse.) A preliminary survey in Seattle shows that 70 percent of such men and women may desire help in changing this pattern. Depression may be an important factor in such cases, and caregivers should be alert to signs of suicidal intent.

The AIDS Prevention Project

The AIDS Prevention Project provides two services to its clients: information and confidential or anonymous clinical assessment. Information is available weekdays from 8 a.m. to 5 p.m. and Wednesdays until 8 p.m. through the AIDS Hotline (206-587-4999). Callers also can make appointments to visit our AIDS resource library to review articles, periodicals, brochures, books, videotapes and audiotapes. We maintain an AIDS slide bank for speakers and operate a speakers' bureau. Additionally, we have developed and tested a high school curriculum and have other curricula available for review.

The AIDS Assessment Clinic provides clinical evaluations and risk reduction counseling to persons at high risk for HIV infection: sexually active gay men, IV drug abusers, and prostitutes and their sexual partners. (Hemophiliacs, another group with high disease prevalence, generally already have knowledgeable health care providers to advise and evaluate them.) The clinic is open weekdays and some evenings and is staffed by two nurse practitioners, four public health advisers and a medical director. Appointments can be arranged through the hotline. Clients are offered a directed history, physical exam, HIV antibody testing, sexually transmitted disease screening, and tuberculosis skin testing. We are especially interested in clients' histories of sexually transmitted disease, sexual practices, and symptoms or signs that suggest HIV infection. Seropositive persons are offered a more detailed exam and a complete blood count. In accord with the aforementioned principles, testing is voluntary and includes appropriate pre- and post-test counseling. These discussions, including clinical assessment and risk-reduction counseling, take approximately an hour.

Clients are offered participation in various research studies, depending on their risk group. We presently are enrolling men who have sex with other men into a longitudinal cohort study to demonstrate changes at six-month intervals in AIDS knowledge, attitudes, behaviors and seroprevalence. These men also are eligible to participate in a study of the oral manifestations of HIV infection. We soon will begin studies in IV drug abusers and prostitutes.

The AIDS Project also performs AIDS surveillance, which includes taking reports of King County residents newly diagnosed with AIDS or with CDC class-IV HIV infection, classifying risk, assessing report completeness and studying the numbers of presumptively diagnosed cases. We also work proactively within the community to lessen the impact of this epidemic by developing efficient care systems and by providing advice to other governmental agencies, to schools and to local businesses.

Evidence of success

Programs for disease control appear to be working. McKusick and others have shown substantial changes in the behaviors of gay men, and DesJarlais has shown a 50-percent reduction in reported needle-sharing and an increased desire for drug treatment among IV drug abusers in New York City. Additionally, data from many metropolitan areas in this country and abroad have shown changes in the frequencies of certain sexually transmitted diseases, including 80-percent reductions in the incidences of rectal gonorrhea, hepatitis, herpes and syphilis among gay men. Among the heterosexually active, the incidence of these diseases is stable or increasing in some areas, which supports the need for more education.

A school AIDS curriculum developed by the AIDS Project produced significant changes in knowledge and attitudes after only one hour of instruction. Public knowledge and attitudes about AIDS also have shown gradual changes. Increasing numbers of AIDS patients in San Francisco and Seattle are dying at home, a trend that attests to the growing success of comprehensive AIDS care programs (Table III).

Summary

To control AIDS and minimize its impact, all health care practitioners must understand and cooperate with public health strategies. Because of the long incubation period from infection to full-blown disease, much time already has been lost, and the effects of today's efforts will take years to materialize. We urge physicians in the Pacific Northwest to get involved in primary, secondary and tertiary disease control. All of us must assist in the education effort; practically all of us will care for persons with AIDS and HIV infections in the years to come. The AIDS epidemic highlights problems with our health care system. Innovative approaches now being developed for AIDS care will benefit all by increasing the general quality, accessibility, efficiency and compassion of that system.

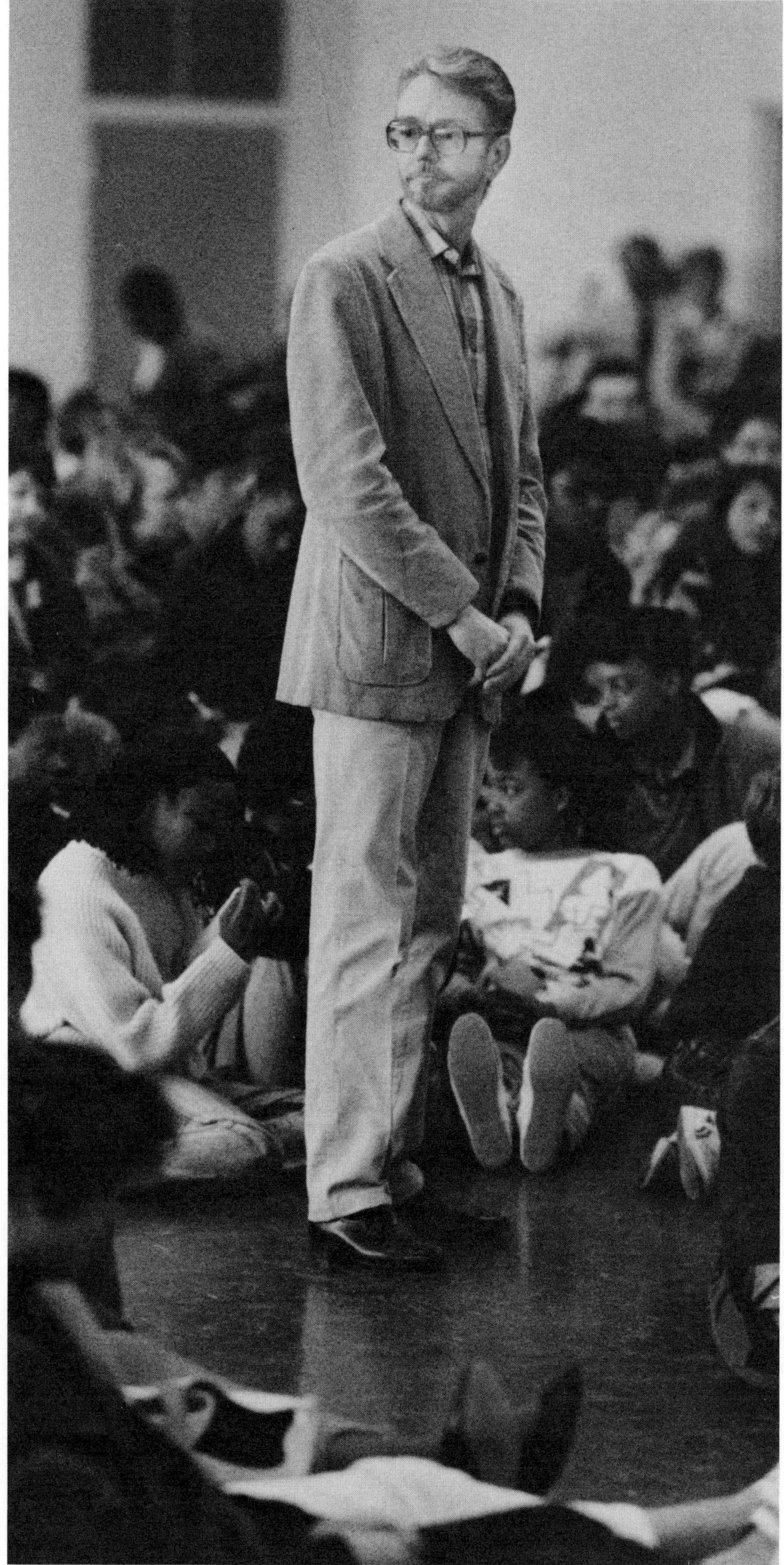

FIGURE 3. Biochemist Allen DeShong, diagnosed as having AIDS in June 1985, talked frankly about his illness with many Seattle school classes before his death in October 1987.

Table III Shifting Sites of Death for Persons with AIDS—Seattle/King County

Place of Death	Number of Deaths (percentage)			
	1983	1984	1985	1986
Home	0	2 (12%)	9 (17%)	22 (28%)
Hospital	3 (75%)	14 (88%)	44 (81%)	53 (67%)
Nursing Home	0	0	0	1 (1%)
Unknown	1 (25%)	0	1 (2%)	2 (3%)
Total	4	16	54	78

Additional Reading

DesJarlais, D.C., Friedman, S.R., Hopkins, W. 1985. Risk reduction for AIDS among IV drug users. *Ann Int Med* 103:755-759.

Fox, R., Odaka, N., Polk, B.F. Effect of learning HTLV-III/LAV antibody status on subsequent sexual activity. Presented at Paris AIDS Conference, June 1986; abstracts p. 167.

Handsfield, H.H. Gonorrhea as a safe-sex indicator in homosexual men. AIDS Quarterly Report; 4th quarter 1986; Seattle-King County Department of Public Health; p. 8.

McKusick, L., Wiley, J.A., Coates, T.J. *et al.* 1985. Reported changes in the sexual behavior of men at risk for AIDS, San Francisco, 1982-1984: The AIDS behavioral research project. *Public Health Reports* 100:622-629.

Owen, W. F. 1980. The clinical approach to the homosexual patient. *Ann Int Med* 93:90-92.

Research and Decisions Corp. A report on: designing an effective AIDS prevention campaign strategy for San Francisco: Results from the second probability study of an urban gay male community. June 28, 1985. 375 Sutter Street, Suite 300, San Francisco, CA 94108.

Zones, J.S., Beeson, D.R., Echenberg, D.F. *et al.* Personal and social consequences of AIDS antibody testing and notification in a cohort of gay and bisexual men. Presented at Paris AIDS Conference, June 1986; abstracts p. 163.

Human Immunodeficiency Viruses and Related Simian AIDS Retroviruses

by Robert W. Coombs, M.D., Ph.D., and Michael G. Katze, Ph.D.

Retroviruses have been implicated as important animal pathogens for more than 60 years. However, retroviruses were identified as etiologic agents in human disease only in the past decade. In this article, we will define a retrovirus; describe in particular the human immunodeficiency retrovirus (HIV); describe the physiopathology of HIV infection; and outline a potential non-human primate model for HIV infection currently under study at the University of Washington.

Retrovirus definition and classification

The family *Retroviridiae* is a large group of ubiquitous viruses that infect all classes of vertebrates. Retroviruses are named for a unique, viral-encoded enzyme called reverse transcriptase. In a reverse of the normal flow of information from DNA to RNA, reverse transcriptase makes a DNA copy of the single-stranded viral RNA genome; hence the prefix "retro." Retroviruses are characterized morphologically by their electron microscopic appearance and by their genomic, antigenic and physiopathologic characteristics.

Although many retroviruses can cause cytopathology in their host cells, most replicate without killing the infected cell. A persistent infection may result, or the infected cell may be transformed and a malignancy induced. Based on these characteristics, human retroviruses are divided into two subfamilies: the transforming oncoviruses and the cytopathic lentiviruses.

While differing in both morphology and physiopathology, these two human retrovirus groups share the following characteristics:

—They bud from the cell surface;

—They have an external envelope containing a large molecular-weight, external receptor-glycoprotein and a smaller, anchoring, transmembrane glycoprotein;

—They possess a high molecular-weight, single-stranded RNA genome;

—They have internal structural proteins that surround the RNA genome;

—They encode an RNA-dependent DNA polymerase (reverse transcriptase).

Retroviruses replicate by a double-stranded DNA intermediate known as a provirus. It often integrates into the host cell's genome but also may take an extrachromosomal, circular form. In addition

Dr. Coombs is a senior fellow in the virology division of the University of Washington Department of Laboratory Medicine. Dr. Katze is a core staff scientist at the UW Regional Primate Research Center and is a UW assistant professor of microbiology.

to reverse transcriptase, at least two host cell polymerases are required; a DNA-dependent DNA polymerase for making multiple copies of the intermediate provirus DNA, and an RNA polymerase II for transcribing the retrovirus proviral DNA into messenger RNA (mRNA). The general scheme for human retrovirus replication is shown in Figure 1.

Oncoviruses

Oncoviruses cause many animal malignancies and characteristically may immortalize cells *in vitro*. In humans the prototype oncoviruses are the human T-cell lymphotropic viruses (HTLV) type I and type II. HTLV-I causes adult T-cell leukemia and may be linked to the degenerative central nervous system disease, tropical spastic paraparesis. HTLV-II has been isolated from some patients with hairy cell leukemia. HTLV-I has CD4+ cell (for example, helper/inducer T-cell or T4 cell) tropism that results in both a direct, *in-vitro* cytopathic effect (syncytia formation with multinucleated giant cells) and in uncontrolled proliferation, causing leukemia *in vivo*, with subsequent immunosuppression and susceptibility to opportunistic infection. These events may occur after decades of latency if the infection was acquired early in childhood or after only a few years if the infection was acquired in adulthood.

The seroprevalence of HTLV-I and -II in the United States is unknown but presumably very small. However, in a study of intravenous drug abusers in Queens, N.Y., the prevalences of serum antibodies to HTLV-I and -II were 9 percent and 18 percent, respectively. Dual infection with HTLV-I or -II and with HIV was found in 27 percent of black intravenous drug abusers from the same area. The impact of this "double jeopardy" on the expression of either HTLV- or HIV-induced disease is unknown but worrisome.

Lentiviruses

The lentivirus subfamily of retroviruses causes slowly progressive diseases with lymphotropic and neurotropic features in both man and ungulates (horses, sheep, cattle and goats). These viruses can produce cytopathology in their target cells, including syncytia formation *in vitro*. The only known members of the human lentivirus group belong to the human immunodeficiency viruses, the etiologic agents of AIDS. These viruses have a tropism for CD4+ T-cells and other cells with the CD4 receptor. The HIV group is much more diverse than previously thought. Two types have been defined: HIV-1 (formerly HTLV-III, LAV-1 and ARV); and HIV-2 (formerly LAV-2). Importantly, a comparison of their genome se-

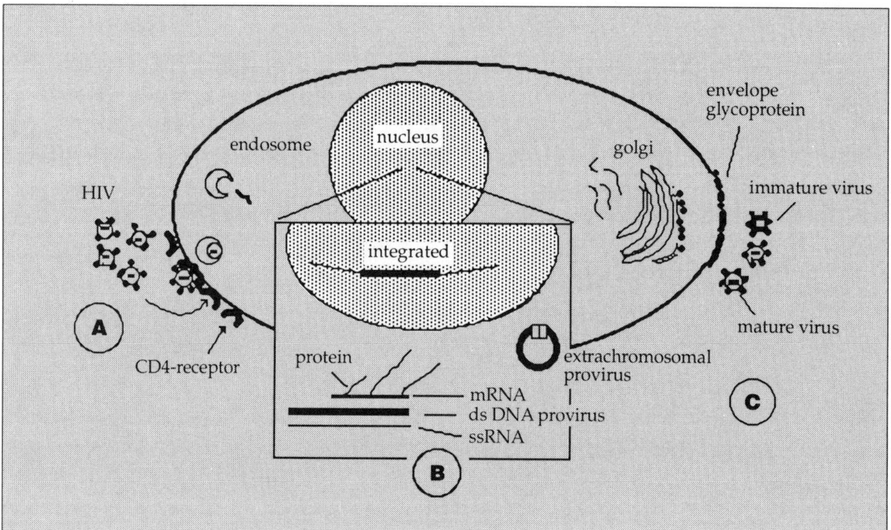

FIGURE 1. Human immunodeficiency virus replication cycle.

(A) *Attachment and Penetration.* The virus attaches to the CD4 receptor by the viral gp120 *env* protein and enters the cell by endocytosis. Fusion of the virus envelope with the endosome releases the virus core that contains the single-stranded RNA genome and reverse transcriptase enzyme.

(B) *Replication.* The reverse transcriptase makes a DNA copy of the RNA genome and the resulting double-stranded DNA provirus either integrates into the host genome or remains extrachromosomal. Transcription of the HIV DNA copy into messenger RNA is then followed by translation of mRNA to viral protein. Several accessory control genes are responsible for regulating viral expression at this stage.

(C) *Assembly.* Viral *env* glycoprotein incorporates into the host cell membrane and serves as a condensation site for the nucleocapsid. The viral particles then bud from the cell surface and the virus core undergoes further extracellular condensation to form the morphologically mature virion.

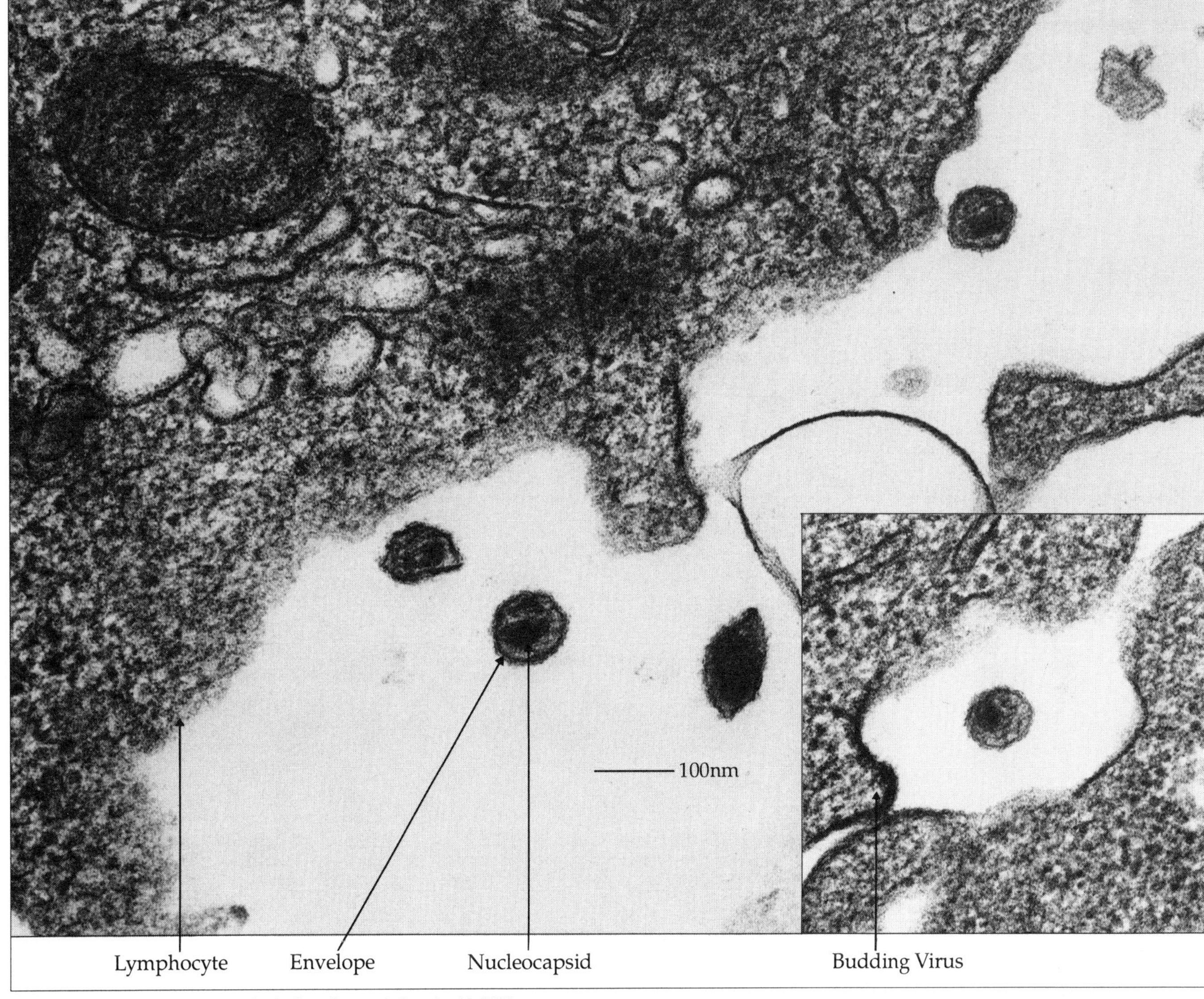

FIGURE 2. An electron micrograph of a lymphocyte infected with HIV.

quences has shown HIV-2 to be distinct from HIV-1. A third HIV isolate, HTLV-IV, has not been fully characterized but appears closely related or identical to the simian immunodeficiency virus and has called into question the independent origin of the two viruses. In addition, there is only limited immunological cross-reactivity between the antigens of HIV-1 currently detected in commercial ELISA and Western blot serologic tests, and the corresponding antigens of HIV-2. For these reasons, current serologic screening tests for HIV-1 cannot reliably detect antibodies to HIV-2. HIV-1 and HIV-2 are placed in the lentivirus group because of morphology, genome organization and protein structure.

Morphology

HIV and the other lentiviruses are morphologically distinct from HTLV-I and HTLV-II. All the retroviruses have a glycoprotein-studded envelope and are approximately 100 nm in size. The conical nucleocapsid core contains the single-stranded RNA genome, structural proteins, and reverse transcriptase. Figure 2 is an electron micrograph of an HIV-infected cell.

Genome organization and protein structure

The genes of HIV and the proteins they encode are important in pathogenesis, are the potential targets for new antiviral drugs, and are of great importance in understanding the current basis for serodiagnosis and recent developments in vaccine research. The genes coding for the major structural (that is, non-regulatory) proteins of HIV are arranged in the left-to-right (5′→3′) direction and are designated *gag*, *pol* and *env* (Figure 3). These genes are flanked by the regulatory-integration sequences in the duplicated long terminal repeat (LTR) segments. In addition, four accessory genes regulate viral expression and infectivity, although the process is not yet understood.

One of these accessory genes, designated 3′-*orf*, apparently has a negative effect on HIV replication and may help to keep HIV latent. The other three accessory genes are necessary for virus production and infectivity. The "*trans*-acting transcriptional" (*tat*III) gene is a split gene flanking the *env* gene. (Note: A gene product is said to act in *trans* when it regulates another gene.) This gene product up-regulates both HIV transcription and translation, and can be considered autostimulatory. Another accessory split-gene flanking the *env* gene is the "anti-repression *trans*-activator" (*art*) gene. The gene is also termed "*trans*-regulator of splicing" (*trs*) because it presumably regulates mRNA splicing. The fourth accessory gene, *sor*, is apparently necessary for the normal infectivity of HIV, although how it does this is unknown. An eighth gene, "R," has an unknown function.

The proteins encoded by the HIV genome identified thus far are: structural core proteins (*gag*); protease, reverse transcriptase, and endonuclease-integrase (*pol*); short open reading frame (*sor*); *trans*-regulatory proteins (*tat*III and *art*/*trs*); envelope glycoproteins (*env*); and the 3′ open reading frame (3′-*orf*).

To summarize, HIV replication requires complex modulation of both transcription and translation; splicing of the mRNA; proteolytic cleavage of the *gag* and *env* polypeptides, and addition of sugar residues (glycosylation) to form the proteins that compose the mature virion.

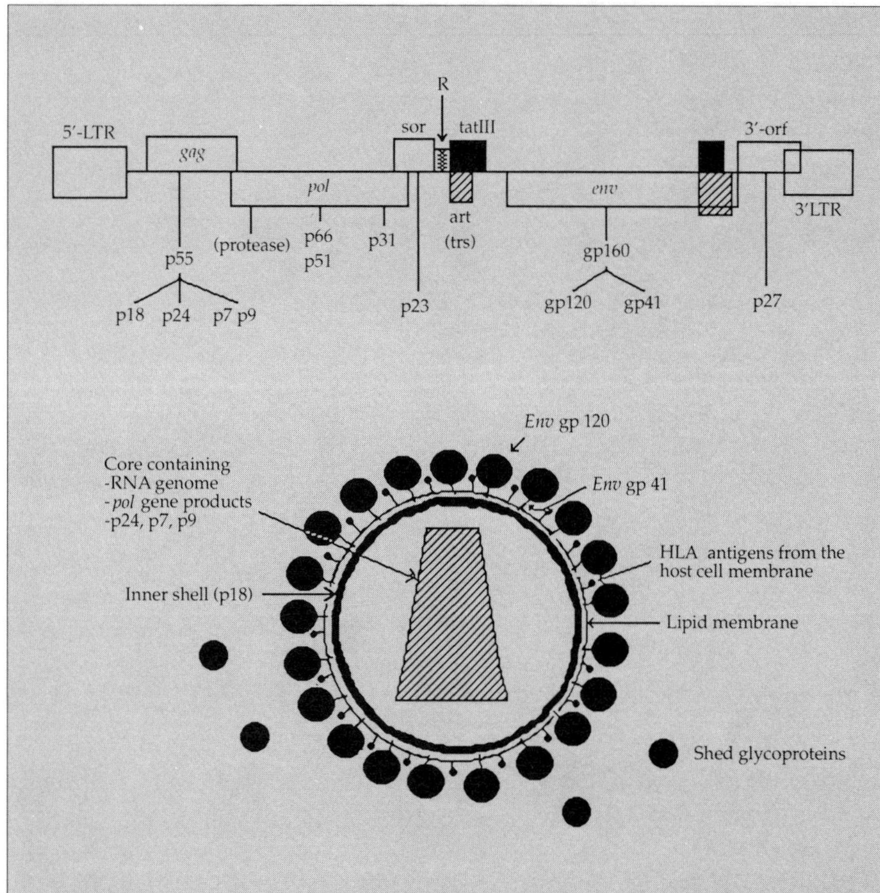

FIGURE 3. The structure of the human immunodeficiency virus type-1 genome. The genes for the structural proteins are designated *gag*, *pol* and *env*. The accessory genes necessary for controlling virus replication and infectivity are *sor*, *tat*III, *art*/*trs*, and *3'-orf*. An eighth gene, "R," has a currently unknown function. The duplicate long terminal repeats (LTR) contain recognition sequences required for integration into the host-cell genome, an inducible host-cell transcription factor, and the regulatory *tat* III protein. The major translational products and their locations in the mature virion also are shown.

The physiopathology of HIV infection: Pathogenesis

The consequences of retrovirus infection reflect a precarious balance between the invading retrovirus, its tropism for specific cells and tissues, and human host resistance. The physiopathologic model of HIV infection can be approached by understanding viral mechanisms of infection, persistence, latency, cell injury, and immune system evasion and modulation. Some aspects of this model are shared by other RNA and DNA viruses, while other aspects are unique to the retrovirus group.

Viral entry into the host

HIV transmission requires either parenteral or intimate mucous membrane exposure to the virus. Transmission by fomites is unlikely, because HIV as an enveloped virus is very sensitive to several envelope-disruptive forces of the environment such as high temperatures, surface tension (for example, drying) and detergents. The concentration of virus in body fluids to which a person is exposed—for example, the small number of infectious HIV particles in saliva vs. the large number in blood—is a very important determinant of transmission. Secretory IgA from the infected host may restrict HIV salivary transmission, as 70 percent of AIDS patients have salivary IgA against the *env*

proteins. The precise mechanisms of transmission are not yet well understood and an animal model system is needed for further study.

Target-cell tropism and virus-receptor interactions

Susceptible cells are required for the process of adsorption, penetration and uncoating. For HIV, the CD4 antigen (that is, T4 or related antigen) is the specific virus receptor. This receptor is a 62-kilodalton glycoprotein that characterizes the CD4 helper/inducer lymphocyte subset. The HIV gp120 *env* binds specifically to the CD4 receptor. HIV infection is associated with a complete loss of CD4 antigen on infected T-cells, and their ultimate death results in a decreased T4/T8 ratio.

The CD4 T-cell is not the only cell type infected by HIV. Other cells, such as the monocyte-macrophage, are CD4+ and probably disseminate HIV to target organs and serve as a reservoir for viral persistence—a feature shared with some other lentiviruses. However, other permissive and semi-permissive cells can be infected, including B lymphocytes positive for Epstein-Barr virus, endothelial cells from established Kaposi's sarcoma, promyelocytes and proerythrocytes, Langerhans cells of the skin, follicular dendritic cells, and several others, some of which do not

express the CD4 antigen. Brain infection with HIV appears to be associated with a mononuclear inflammatory infiltrate, although some evidence exists for infection of primary central nervous system cells that may express a CD4-related antigen.

Genomic diversity

Within the *env* gene, localized regions of extraordinary hypervariability are interspersed with well-conserved (nonvariable) regions. The conserved regions probably encode for the CD4 attachment site. The degree of variability in the *env* gene is unique to the lentivirus group. The mechanism of variation may be due to errors in reverse transcription leading to substitutions and misreading. The mutation rate in the *env* gene is 1 million times greater than that of DNA viruses and 10 to 100 times greater than that of other retroviruses. This extraordinary *env* gene hypervariability corresponds to amino acid changes of as much as 20 percent among divergent HIV-1 isolates. It may modify several biologic properties, including tissue tropism, virulence, replication rate and sensitivity to antiviral chemotherapy, and it may allow the virus to evade the immune response.

Latency and persistence

For any virus infection to persist, viral gene expression must be restricted. Three patterns of restricted viral expression are known:

—Latent infection, characterized by intermittent episodes of acute disease with no virus detected between episodes (for example, oral-labial or genital herpes simplex virus);

—Chronic infection, in which the virus is always demonstrable but disease is absent (for example, cytomegalovirus); and

—Persitent infections, characterized by a long incubation period with slowly increasing amounts of transcriptional-translational products and eventually symptomatic disease (for example, subacute sclerosing panencephalitis from measles virus infection).

The lentiviruses—HIV in particular—share features from all three patterns, but are best described as persistent infections.

The HIV provirus integrates randomly in the infected host cell genome, but most provirus DNA remains extrachromosomal. The degree of viral transcription and translation depends on the infected CD4+ cell's stage of differentiation. That stage, in turn, is probably related to exogenous antigen stimulation. (That is, exogenous antigen stimulation may promote HIV-1 replication.) Integration of human retroviruses differs from that of certain other animal retroviruses in that no transforming genes (oncogenes) are associated with the viral genome, and the proviral genome is not regularly inserted next to a host transforming gene. Provirus integration is important not only in defining the pathologic mechanisms of the retrovirus group *per se*, but it also suggests that current chemotherapeutic interventions directed against actively replicating virus will not "cure" cells latently infected with HIV proviral DNA.

Mechanisms of cytopathology

A dilemma in understanding HIV physiopathology is the mechanism by which the CD4+ T-cell population is depleted when only 1 in 10,000 to 1 in 100,000 T-cells appear to be infected. The mechanism of CD4+ cell depletion is complex and poorly understood. It may be a function of both cell fusion and an autoimmune interaction against the CD4 receptor triggered by the shedding of *env* glycoprotein from infected cells. The CD4 antigen, in addition to being the HIV receptor, directly participates *in vitro* in cell fusion between infected and uninfected CD4+ cell lines. Introducing HIV *env* glycoprotein into the infected cell membrane destabilizes the membrane and probably causes cytoskeletal alterations in the microtubules, microfilaments and intermediate filaments that are required for syncytia formation, viral assembly, budding and release. The cytopathic feature of HIV

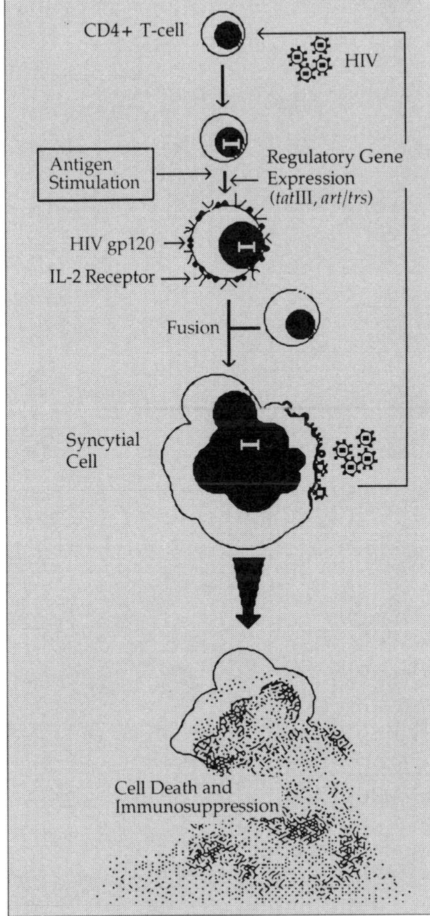

FIGURE 4. Proposed dependence of HIV expression on the antigenic stimulation of infected CD4+ T-cells (after Zagury, 1986). Following antigen stimulation of the latently infected CD4+ T-cell, HIV is expressed through complex and incompletely understood mechanisms involving the *tat*III and *art/trs* regulatory genes. Infected cells expressing viral envelope glycoprotein (gp120) and interleukin-2 (IL-2) receptors fuse with uninfected CD4+ cells, form syncytia, express virus, and then die in an accelerated fashion. This eventually produces an immunodeficiency that usually progresses to AIDS. In the absence of suitable antigenic stimulation, HIV probably remains latent in the infected CD4+ T-cell.

appears to reside in the amino terminus of the transmembrane glycoprotein gp41. It thus appears that infection in one CD4 cell causes agglutination and fusion of other uninfected cells, leading to their subsequent dysfunction and destruction.

Zagury *et al* recently proposed a model for HIV infection (Figure 4). The major features of this model are:

—HIV replication may be promoted by repeated rounds of antigenic stimulation *in vivo* (for example, by concurrent infection with other viruses, bacteria, fungi and protozoans; and by exposure to allogenic cells such as semen and blood).

—Successive cycles of HIV latency and expression result from fine-tuning of the regulatory *tat*III and *art/trs* genes. In turn, *env* and *gag* mRNAs accumulate, followed by a burst of viral replication, leading to cell death with depletion of the CD4+ T-cell population, and subsequent immunosuppression.

Support for this model comes from recent observations that herpes simplex virus type 1 can activate transcription of latent HIV, and that antigenic stimulation of HIV-infected T-cells results in the expression of an inducible, cell-associated transcription factor that activates latent HIV.

Based on these *in-vitro* observations, it is reasonable to advise HIV-seropositive patients to modify their high-risk sexual and/or intravenous drug-abusing practices and to avoid further immune system stimulation either by direct foreign antigen exposure (for example, semen and blood) or by sexually and parenterally transmitted infectious agents.

Immunopathogenesis

As mentioned above, lymphotropic infection by human and lower primate retroviruses characteristically results in immunosuppression. In the case of HIV infection, selective failure of both adaptive immunity (depletion of the CD4+ helper-inducer subset of lymphocytes) and natural immunity (large granular lymphocytes) results in the immune imbalance. Such imbalance leaves the patient susceptible to several opportunistic infections and malignancies. The CD4+ lymphocyte population normally represents approximately 60 percent of T-cells and contains effectors for delayed hypersensitivity as well as inducers for killer T-cell generation, B-cell differentiation into immunoglobulin-secreting plasma cells, and active suppressor-cell development. This contrasts to the CD8+ population, which is not infected by HIV. The CD8+ subset normally represents approximately 30 percent of the T-cells and contains effectors for killer T-cells and other cells that suppress cell-mediated reactivities and immunoglobulin production.

The functional T-cell defects produced by HIV infection result in decreased lymphokines (IL-2) and decreased helper-inducer functions for other T- and B-cells, while the defect in the large granular lymphocytes results in decreased alpha-interferon production. *In vitro*, the CD8+ T-cell

suppresses viral expression by infected CD4+ T-cells. The B-lymphocyte defects result in a decreased antibody response to soluble antigens with concomitant polyclonal elevation of serum immunoglobulins, primarily of the IgG and IgA classes; this stimulation may represent a complex set of interactions involving HIV itself, Epstein-Barr virus, or possibly the newly recognized herpes-like lymphotropic virus. The monocyte defects may result in the spontaneous increase in interleukin-1 secretion (hence, the observed fever with this disease) and possibly tumor necrosis factor (hence, the wasting component of AIDS, although this may be much more complex, with superimposed gastrointestinal infections and malabsorption). A direct immunosuppressive role for HIV *env* or *gag* proteins has not been demonstrated.

A perplexing feature of HIV infection is that HIV persists in lymphocytes and plasma despite antibody production. Neutralizing antibody binds to HIV gp120 *env* and is found in most patients with AIDS and AIDS-related complex (ARC). Although these antibodies reportedly block attachment of the virus *in vitro*, it is not known whether this confers immunity *in vivo*. Escape from antibody neutralization may reflect direct cell-to-cell transmission of the virus, a changing antigen expression of the envelope glycoprotein due to hypervariability in the *env* gene, or both. Clearly, an animal model is required to study the mechanisms by which HIV escapes the immune system.

SAIDS-D and SIV primate retroviruses

Historically, animal models have proved invaluable in studying the pathogenesis of human viral diseases. Studies using non-human primates often have paved the way for life-saving vaccines, with poliovirus the classic example. No successful animal model has been described thus far for the human immunodeficiency viruses. Chimpanzees are the only animals susceptible to HIV infection, but infected chimpanzees show no clinical symptoms of an immunosuppressive disease, and not enough chimpanzees are available for the necessary studies. For these reasons, the University of Washington Regional Primate Research Center is making a major effort to develop an animal model for AIDS-like diseases in non-human primates. A brief summary of our efforts follows.

SAIDS-D virus

We have observed an acquired immunodeficiency syndrome in various macaques that is similar in certain respects to human AIDS. A novel type-D retrovirus, distinct from previously mentioned viruses (human retroviruses are type C), was isolated by cocultivating explants of fibromatous tissue obtained from naturally infected rhesus monkeys (*Macaca mulatta*). Monkeys infected with this virus, termed SAIDS-D/Washington, show an immunodeficiency syndrome characterized by persistent diarrhea, progressive weight loss, anemia, lymphocytopenia, unusual chronic infections, and a peculiar fibromatous tumor called retroperitoneal fibromatosis. Immunohistochemical studies have shown factor VIII-related antigen in endothelial and fibroblast-like cells throughout the retroperitoneal fibromatosis lesions similar to that described for Kaposi's sarcoma. Thus, in its progressive form, SAIDS-D causes lymphoid depletion, opportunistic infections and an unusual neoplasm (retroperitoneal fibromatosis). No cross-reactivity was found between SAIDS-D virus and the human lentiviruses at either the protein or the nucleic acid level.

SIV virus

We have isolated a lentivirus from the malignant lymphoma of a 6-year-old male macaque *Macaca nemestrina*. This simian lentivirus, called SIV for simian immunodeficiency virus, is partially related to the human lentiviruses—HIV-1 and HIV-2—isolated from AIDS patients. Similar but non-identical simian immunodeficiency viruses have been isolated at other regional primate centers. Serological analyses reveal that antisera from sick macaques react strongly with HIV core proteins, but only weakly with the envelope glycoproteins. Conversely, antisera from seropositive AIDS patients show cross-reactivity with SIV core antigens. The *in-vitro* growth characteristics of SIV also are similar to HIV: SIV is tropic for CD4+ T-cells and its infectivity can be blocked by anti-CD4 antibodies.

When healthy rhesus monkeys were experimentally infected with SIV, an AIDS-like immunosuppressive disease was induced that often led to death. The animals developed diarrhea and lost as much as 60 percent of their body weight. The absolute number of CD4+ T-cells in their peripheral blood lymphocytes fell to one-half normal as early as two weeks following infection. Since the number of circulating CD8+ T-cells remained unchanged, the CD4/CD8 ratio decreased in the infected monkeys. However, recent studies at the University of Washington show that some monkeys terminally ill with SIV have dramatically reduced numbers of both CD4 and CD8 cells. We also have found a large increase in the percentage of B-cells in infected animals.

Future studies at the UW Regional Primate Research Center

Considerable work remains to precisely define the nature of SAIDS-D and SIV and the diseases these viruses produce in macaques. It is clear, however, that both viruses—particularly SIV—provide excellent models with features analogous to retrovirus infec-tions in humans. We have initiated major studies of SAIDS-D and SIV that focus on: (1) natural and experimental transmission of both viruses, (2) transmission of SIV from infected mothers to the fetus or newborn, (3) development of both SAIDS-D and SIV vaccines, (4) testing of antiviral drugs to block SAIDS-D and SIV retroviral infection, and (5) development of monoclonal antibodies against SAIDS-D and SIV for both diagnostic and basic research purposes. Our long-range goal is to study the gene expression of both viruses at the molecular level and to compare the simian AIDS viruses to the human AIDS viruses.

The issues involved in questions of SIV-HIV relatedness at the nucleic acid level, and whether the former has given rise to the latter, are clouded at press time. The SIV group of viruses apparently may have more homology with HIV-2 than with HIV-1. Nevertheless, a careful, detailed molecular analysis of the virus groups is needed before any definitive statements can be made about the origins of human AIDS.

Summary

There are two major subfamilies of retroviruses that infect humans: oncoviruses, represented by HTLV-I and -II; and lentiviruses, represented by the human immunodeficiency virus (HIV) group. Lentiviruses are characterized by their ability to infect and kill the CD4+ lymphocyte, which inverts the CD4+/CD8+ lymphocyte ratio and causes an immune imbalance that leads to the opportunistic infections and malignancies characteristic of AIDS. The progression of this persistent virus infection may depend on the antigenic stimulation and subsequent differentiation of the infected CD4+ cell.

The basic mechanism of CD4+ cell depletion cannot be attributed to HIV infection of every CD4+ cell. It likely arises from a combination of cell fusion between infected and uninfected CD4+ cells and from autoimmune destruction of CD4+ cells triggered by the interaction of shed viral glycoprotein with the CD4+ receptor on uninfected cells.

Hypervariability in the HIV *env* gene probably confers corresponding antigenic variability in envelope glycoproteins. The consequences of this hypervariability could include development of strains resistant to new chemotherapeutic agents and/or to the immune response produced by natural infection or by candidate vaccines. An animal model of simian immunodeficiency virus under study at the UW may help to elucidate the physiopathologic mechanisms of HIV infection in man and facilitate the development of successful antiviral drugs and viral vaccines.

Additional Reading

Gallo, R.C. and Wong-Staal, F. 1985. A human T-lymphotropic retrovirus (HTLV-III) as the cause of the aquired immunodeficiency syndrome. *Ann Intern Med* 103:679-689.

Gallo, R.C. 1987. The AIDS retrovirus. *Sci Amer* 256:47-56.

Gallo, R.C. 1986. The first human retrovirus. *Sci Amer* 255:88-98.

Haase, A.T. 1986. Pathogenesis of lentivirus infections. *Nature* 322:130-136.

Weiss, A., Hollander, H. and Stobo, J. 1985. Acquired immunodeficiency syndrome: epidemiology, virology, and immunology. *Ann Rev Med* 36:545-562.

Zagury, D., Bernard, J., Leonard, R., Cheynier, R. *et al.* 1986. Long-term cultures of HTLV-III-infected T cells: a model of cytopathology of T-cell depletion in AIDS. *Science* 231:850-853.

Adams, S.W. 1987. Simian T-lymphotropic viruses. *Lab Animal* 16:33-39.

Laboratory Diagnosis of Human Immunodeficiency Virus Infection

by Lynn Goldstein, M.D., and Robert Coombs, M.D., Ph.D.

Persons infected with the human immunodeficiency virus (HIV)[1] are usually identified by the presence of antibody reactive with the retrovirus. Virus can be isolated from the majority of HIV-seropositive individuals.

It is fairly easy to arrive at a clinical suspicion of acquired immunodeficiency syndrome (AIDS) given the appropriate signs and symptoms and a history of membership in a high-risk group for HIV infection: a homosexual/bisexual male; an intravenous drug abuser; a recipient of multiple blood product transfusions; those having heterosexual contact with a high-risk or HIV-seropositive partner; a native of certain areas of Africa or Haiti; a male or female prostitute; or a child born to parents who are members of these risk groups.

Physicians face a major challenge in diagnosing HIV infection in a person who is asymptomatic, who has atypical signs and symptoms, or who denies membership in a high-risk group. Current clinical and laboratory approaches to the diagnosis of HIV infection are outlined in Table I. For descriptive and technical purposes, laboratory detection of HIV infection can be stratified as first, second and third-generation tests.

First-generation HIV tests: Enzyme immunoassays

Enzyme immunoassays were first developed to detect HIV antibodies in infected potential blood donors. These tests have now been adopted for screening high-risk groups for HIV infections. Following the initial screening procedure, more specific tests confirm the diagnosis.

To understand the basis for serologic testing, a brief review of the HIV antigens is helpful. HIV has three major structural genes—*gag*, *pol* and *env*—each of which codes for one or more proteins expressed in infected cells or in the mature virus (see "Human Immunodeficiency Viruses and Related Simian AIDS Retroviruses" on page 16). The *gag* gene encodes the major core proteins, including p55, a polypeptide of 55 kilodaltons, which is cleaved to form p24 and p18. The *pol* gene encodes three

Table I Detection of Human Immunodeficiency Virus Infection

1. Immunological Abnormalities
   —Not specific or sensitive
   —Opportunistic infections are highly specific indicators for HIV infection when other recognized causes of immunodeficiency are absent

2. Clinical Abnormalities Typical of HIV Infection
   —Not sensitive
   —Indirect evidence for HIV infection
   —Define cases for epidemiologic surveillance

3. Serologic Response (Enzyme Immunoassay)
   —Widely available and the primary diagnostic test
   —Defined sensitivity and specificity
   —Sensitivity and specificity may be improved with recombinant viral proteins and synthetic peptides
   —Positive predictive value varies with prevalence of HIV infection in the population and usually requires confirmatory testing by Western blot, immunofluorescence or radioimmunoprecipitation

4. Antigen Detection
   —Investigational
   —Undefined sensitivity and specificity for clinical specimens
   —Solid phase radioimmunoassay and enzyme immunoassay antigen capture usually detect 30 picograms of p24 antigen/ml of serum

5. Viral Genome Detection by Hybridization
   —Investigational
   —.01–0.001 percent of CD4+ T-cells are positive for HIV RNA
   —Undefined sensitivity and specificity
   —Sensitivity may be improved by *in-vitro* enzymatic amplification of the HIV genome

6. Virus Culture
   —Still primarily a research procedure
   —Viral replication is followed by measurement of viral products
   —Undefined sensitivity but highly specific

proteins: p66 and p51, both known to have reverse transcriptase activity, and the nuclease/integrase p31. The *env* gene encodes a glycoprotein of 160 kilodaltons, gp160, which is cleaved into the surface glycoprotein gp120 and the transmembrane protein gp41. HIV-infected persons produce a spectrum of antibodies to all or some of these proteins.

A prototype enzyme immunoassay procedure is shown in Figure 1. The test detects antibodies to multiple viral proteins, since a whole viral lysate is used as the target antigen. Serum samples that the enzyme immunoassay shows to be "initially reactive" are repeat tested in duplicate to rule out technical errors in test performance. If either repeat test is positive, the sample is considered "repeatably reactive." To rule out false-positive enzyme immunoassay results, these reactive specimens are then tested by a confirmatory method.

Clinical studies have shown that the enzyme immunoassay procedure has greater than 99-percent sensitivity and specificity[2] in both blood donor and high-risk popula-

Dr. Goldstein is vice president of research and development at Genetic Systems Corp. in Seattle. Dr. Coombs is a senior fellow in the virology division of the Department of Laboratory Medicine at the University of Washington.

1 This group is expanding and had two fully characterized types at press time: HIV-1 is the major isolate responsible for the world pandemic. HIV-2, distinct from HIV-1, has been isolated from AIDS patients from West Africa. Preliminary reports suggest that "HTLV-IV," the other HIV-isolate from West Africa, is closely related or identical to the simian immunodeficiency virus (SIV). (See "Human Immunodeficiency Viruses and Related Simian AIDS Retroviruses" on page 16.) Throughout this article, "HIV" refers to HIV-1.

2 The sensitivity of the test is defined as the probability that a person who has antibody to HIV will be positive in the test. Specificity is the probability that a person who does not have antibody to HIV will be negative in the test. The predictive value of a positive test is the probability that a person has antibody to HIV when the test is positive.

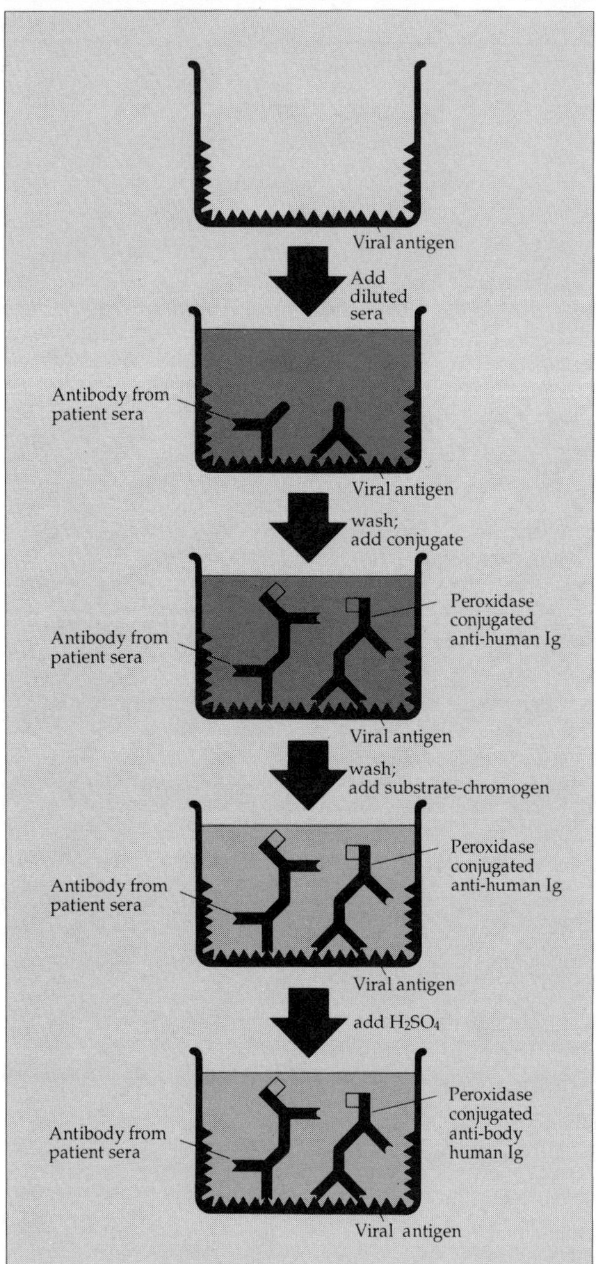

FIGURE 1.

The purified, inactivated virus is adsorbed onto wells of a microwell plate.

Samples to be tested are diluted in sample diluent and added to each well, incubated with the adsorbed antigen and washed. If antibodies to the virus are present, they bind to antigen and are not removed by washing.

The conjugate reagent, peroxidase-labeled goat anti-human immunoglobulin, is then added to the wells and will bind to the antibody-antigen complex, if present. Unbound conjugate is removed by a wash step.

Next, chromogen reagent is added to the plate and allowed to incubate. A blue or blue-green color develops in proportion to the amount of antibody bound to the antigen-coated plate.

The addition of acid stops the enzyme reaction, resulting in a color change to yellow. The optical absorbance of controls and specimens is determined with a spectrophotometer with wavelength set at 450 nm.

tions. The predictive value of a positive result, however, varies with the population tested due to differences in prevalence of the infection in low- and high-risk populations. For example, the Genetic Systems LAV enzyme immunoassay was tested on 9,703 serum and plasma samples from blood donation centers from cities considered both high- and low-risk for HIV infection. In this population, 21 specimens were repeatably reactive and 14 of 21 were positive by a confirmatory method, demonstrating 100-percent sensitivity and 99.9-percent specificity. The predictive value of a positive enzyme immunoassay result in this population with low prevalence (<1 percent) of disease thus was 67 percent. In studies from 1,414 patients from a high-risk group, the sensitivity of the enzyme immunoassay compared with the confirmatory method was 99.9 percent (875 positive/876 confirmatory positive) and the specificity was 99.9 percent (537 nega-

tive/538 confirmatory negative). Since this population had a high prevalence of disease (66 percent), the enzyme immunoassay's positive predictive value was 99.9 percent. In general, it is important to have a bimodal distribution of non-reactive and reactive results (that is, no "grey area" of overlap between reactives and non-reactives) independent of the population tested to achieve maximum sensitivity and specificity in the enzyme immunoassay.

Compared with other test formats, the enzyme immunoassay has the advantages of sensitivity, specificity, and ease of automation for time and cost reductions. Several problems can occur with the procedure, however, that may give false-positive or false-negative results. False-positive results are most often due to reactions to some specific cellular antigens in the cell line used to produce the virus. Circulating antibodies to HLA, nuclear, and other cellular antigens can be seen in patients with autoimmune

disease, lymphoproliferative disorders, in multiparous women, and in people who have received multiple transfusions. False-negative results may be due either to diminished antibody associated with late-stage disease or to the lack of detectable antibody soon after initial infection.

Current enzyme immunoassay screens are designed to detect antibody to HIV-1. They do not reliably detect antibody to HIV-2 in blood from persons with HIV-2 infection because HIV-1 and HIV-2 exhibit antigenic cross-reactivity only between *gag* and *pol* proteins, not between *env* proteins.

Confirmatory tests

Following enzyme immunoassay screening, repeatably reactive specimens are tested by a confirmatory method to assure the specific reaction to the virus. Such methods include those that detect antibody to individual viral proteins, such as Western blot or radioimmunoprecipitation, and those that use infected cultured cells to detect antibody, such as immunofluorescence.

The Western blot, shown in Figure 2, is the most common method used to detect the antibody response to specific HIV viral proteins. Purified HIV viral proteins are electrophoresed in sodium dodecyl sulfate gels and transferred to nitrocellulose paper. The paper is then incubated with the serum sample, and specific antibody is detected with an enzyme-conjugated, anti-human antibody and enzyme substrate. Most human sera that contain antibodies to the virus react with a constellation of viral proteins repres enting envelope (gp120, gp41) or core (p55, p31, p24, p18) or both (lane g, Figure 2). A small percentage of sera reacts only with single core proteins (p24). The specificity of antibodies to a single core protein of HIV and the significance of these reactions is uncertain; therefore, this reaction pattern is called atypical or indeterminant.

The Western blot has demonstrated greater than 99-percent sensitivity and specificity, but the procedure is time-consuming, labor-intensive, and subjective. The method is less sensitive for detection of antibodies to the viral glycoproteins and very sensitive for antibodies to viral core proteins (p24). The Western blot's use to confirm enzyme immunoassay results is important in populations with a low prevalence of infection. In high-risk populations, the predictive value of a positive is greater than 99 percent and a confirmatory method may not be necessary.

Radioimmunoprecipitation is another method that detects antibody to specific viral proteins. HIV viral proteins are radiolabeled with amino acids, and lysates are incubated with the serum sample. Following washing procedures, the radiolabeled proteins binding to the antibodies are electrophoresed on sodium dodecyl sulfate gels and detected by autoradiography. This procedure is less adaptable to a clinical laboratory than the Western blot, but may be more sensitive in detecting viral glycoproteins.

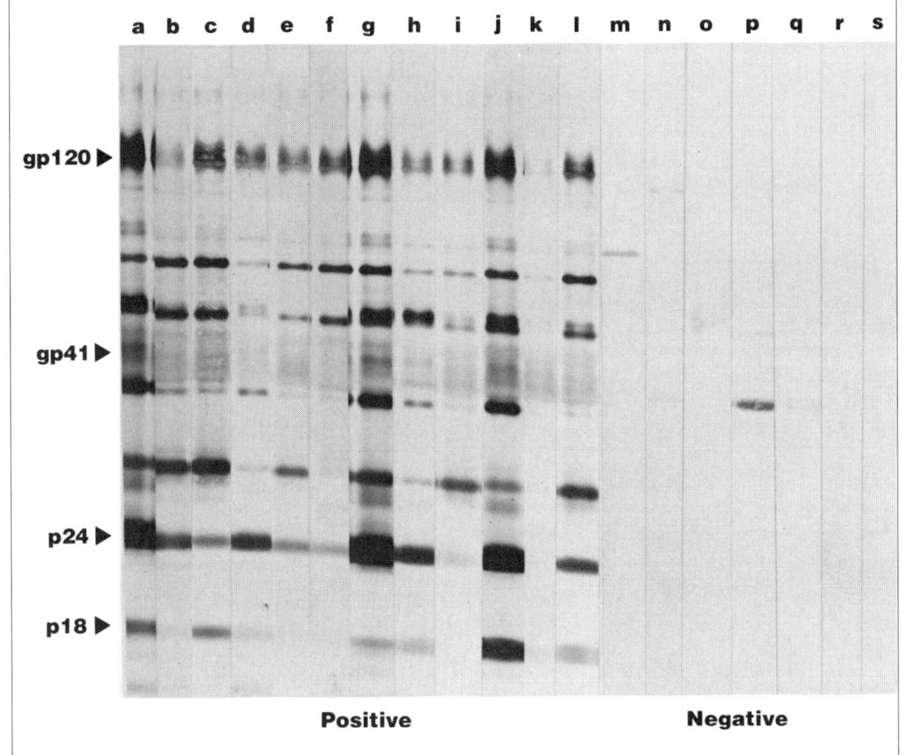

FIGURE 2. Western blot of sera positive and negative for antibody to specific HIV viral proteins. Purified HIV viral proteins are electrophoresed on gels, transferred to paper, and antibody is detected by an enzymatic assay. Sera positive for antibody to HIV react with a constellation of viral proteins representing envelope (gp120, gp41), core (p18, p24) or both, as demonstrated in lanes a-l. Sera negative for antibody to HIV do not react with HIV viral proteins, as demonstrated in lanes m-s.

Immunofluorescence is a third method of detecting HIV antibody. A serum sample is incubated with HIV-infected cells fixed to microscope slides. Specific antibody is detected by fluorescein-labeled, anti-human antibody, and positive cells are visualized using the fluorescence microscope. The method has been demonstrated to be as sensitive and specific as the Western blot in laboratories experienced with this technique. It is relatively simple and inexpensive, but it can be subjective and is not widely available.

Second- and third-generation HIV tests

To develop more sensitive and specific tests for HIV, second-generation assays have used recombinant DNA technology or synthetic peptide chemistry to detect antibodies to specific viral proteins. Viral glycoproteins encoded by the *env* gene (gp41) and core proteins from the *gag* gene (p24) have been expressed in *Escherichia coli* and have been used in enzyme immunoassay and Western blot assay formats. The recombinant proteins from the *env* region have shown greater than 99-percent sensitivity. However, since the antibody response to HIV is diverse, it is important to include viral proteins from both *env* and *gag* gene products. Analysis of recombinants from the *gag* gene show that the immune response has diverse reactivity, in contrast to that in the *env* region. Therefore, recombinants in the *gag* region show approximately 80-percent sensitivity for anti-p24 antibodies compared to Western blot.

An alternative approach is to use chemically synthesized peptides representing immunodominant regions of the viral proteins. Our laboratory and others have shown that a 25-amino-acid sequence from the gp41 protein of the virus has greater than 99-percent sensitivity when compared with enzyme immunoassay and Western blot. Synthetic peptides may be more sensitive and specific than the recombinant proteins because they are not contaminated by bacterial proteins.

Both recombinant proteins and synthetic peptides offer the advantages of cost, safety, and manufacturing reliability. They also may be more sensitive and specific because the target antigens do not contain cellular contaminants present in many enzyme immunoassay tests that use whole viral lysates. In addition, individual viral antigens can be used to detect antibody to separate viral proteins. This may be useful in determining the prognosis of seropositive people, since individuals with AIDS-related complex (ARC) and AIDS appear to have a lower titer and lower prevalence of anti-*gag* (p24) antibodies. It has therefore been suggested that absence of anti-*gag* antibodies is associated with poor prognosis.

Third-generation tests have been developed that detect HIV viral antigen. These assays utilize an antigen capture immunoassay format in which specific anti-HIV antibody (monoclonal or polyclonal) is used to capture HIV antigen. Enzyme-labeled, anti-HIV antibody and enzyme substrate are then used to detect the antibody-antigen complex. Current assays detect the p24 core antigen. These tests can be used to detect antigen during viral culture, replacing the tedious method of monitoring for reverse transcriptase, the viral enzyme.

The tests also have been used to detect antigen in serum specimens. Studies show that very early after infection, antigen is present for a short time in the serum before circulating antibody develops. The "window" of antigen ranges from two weeks to two months or more after acquiring infection. Subsequently, more people who have ARC and AIDS have detectable serum p24 antigen than do healthy, seropositive people. The relationship between the presence of p24 antigen, HIV recovery from plasma, and the lower titer of antibody to p24 in patients with AIDS or ARC remains to be determined. Finally, it has been reported that persons treated with the HIV antiviral drug zidovudine (formerly known as azidothymidine or AZT) may

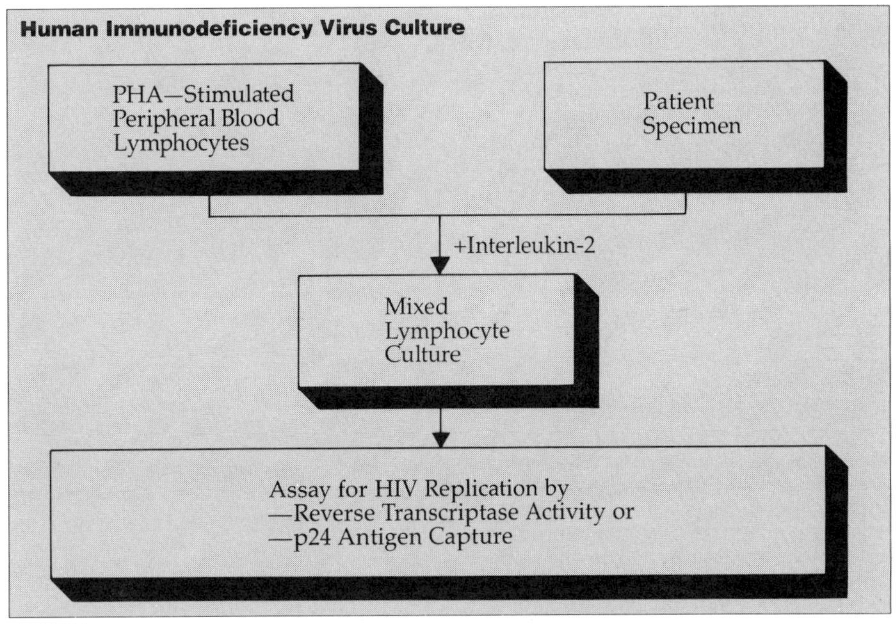

FIGURE 3.

Table II Isolation of HIV from peripheral blood lymphocytes of HIV-seropositive persons—Centers for Disease Control, Atlanta, Georgia

Group	Persons Tested	HIV Culture-Positive	
	N	N	(%)
Asymptomatic (CDC II)			
Blood donors*	16	16	(100)
Homosexual men	31	15	(48)
Hemophiliacs	13	1	(8)
Total	60	32	(53)
Lymphadenopathy (CDC III)			
Blood donors*	6	6	(100)
Homosexual men	31	20	(65)
Hemophiliacs	6	5	(83)
Total	43	31	(72)
AIDS (CDC IV)			
Transfusion recipients	7	7	(100)
Homosexual men	13	12	(92)
Hemophiliacs	4	3	(75)
Total	24	22	(92)

*Implicated in transfusion-associated AIDS

After Francis, D.P. *et al.* 1985. *Ann Int Med* 103:717-722.

show a reduced amount of circulating antigen. The antigen test, therefore, may be useful to monitor patients on antiviral chemotherapy.

DNA probe technology for viral RNA and DNA is an alternative methodology for virus detection. By using various hybridization techniques, HIV sequences can be detected in the peripheral blood lymphocytes or tissues of less than 50 percent of symptomatic, HIV-seropositive patients. (This contrasts to HIV culture, which has a sensitivity of greater than 98 percent.) Moreover, infected cells are observed at a very low frequency—less than 0.01 percent of the total mononuclear cells from the peripheral blood. This difference in sensitivity may be due to a low number of HIV genome copies per cell or to sampling error due to the extremely low frequency of cells expressing HIV. By employing *in-vitro* enzymatic methods to amplify selective parts of the HIV genome (a process called gene amplification) prior to hybridization, the sensitivity of nucleic acid hybridization may approach that of virus culture. The gene amplification method also is amenable to automation and has the potential to decrease both the time and cost of virus culture.

HIV culture

Since the time that both Montagnier and Gallo isolated and subsequently characterized HIV in 1983, many laboratories around the world have isolated HIV from infected individuals with varying success. HIV is isolated in primary mixed-lymphocyte culture (Figure 3). Peripheral blood lymphocytes to be tested for the presence of HIV are separated from heparinized, fresh, whole blood by ficoll-hypaque density gradient centrifugation. The mononuclear cell cushion is removed and cocultivated with phytohemagglutinin (PHA)-stimulated normal peripheral blood lymphocytes from HIV-seronegative donors. The PHA (a plant-derived mitogen) stimulates the normal CD4+ T-cells to produce receptors for the lymphokine interleukin-2 (IL-2). In the presence of purified, exogenous IL-2, the CD4+ T-cells further differentiate into blasts, which are more receptive to virus infection. Traces of PHA and the antigenic stimulation from the allogenic mixed-lymphocyte culture conditions are responsible for stimulating the expression of HIV in the patient's infected CD4+-mononuclear cells. Cultures are assayed for HIV production twice weekly and are incubated for at least 28 days before being considered negative. Other specimens—including serum, plasma, cerebrospinal fluid, genital secretions, and homogenized tissues—are cocultivated with normal donor lymphocytes by a similar procedure.

HIV replicates in culture to a point where viral products can be accurately measured. The two most useful methods for quantitating HIV replication *in vitro* are measurement of reverse transcriptase or p24 antigen in the cell-free culture supernatant. An increase in either viral product over time reflects HIV replication. Because reverse transcriptase also is found in human retroviruses other than HIV—for example, human T-lymphotropic virus types I and II (HTLV-I and -II)—cultures positive for reverse transcriptase activity require confirmation by electron microscopy, immunofluorescence or p24 antigen capture. Production of a characteristic cytopathic effect (multinucleated giant cells) also may be used as a qualitative marker for HIV production. In our laboratory, 80 to 90 percent of HIV-positive peripheral blood lymphocytes are detected by the second week of culture.

Isolation of HIV from different HIV-seropositive populations

HIV has been isolated not only from peripheral blood lymphocytes, but also from a number of clinical specimens including tears, saliva, serum, plasma, breast milk, cerebrospinal fluid, brain, peripheral nerve, skin, semen, cervical secretions, and various internal organs. Although not all of these sources have been implicated in the epidemiologic transmission of infection,

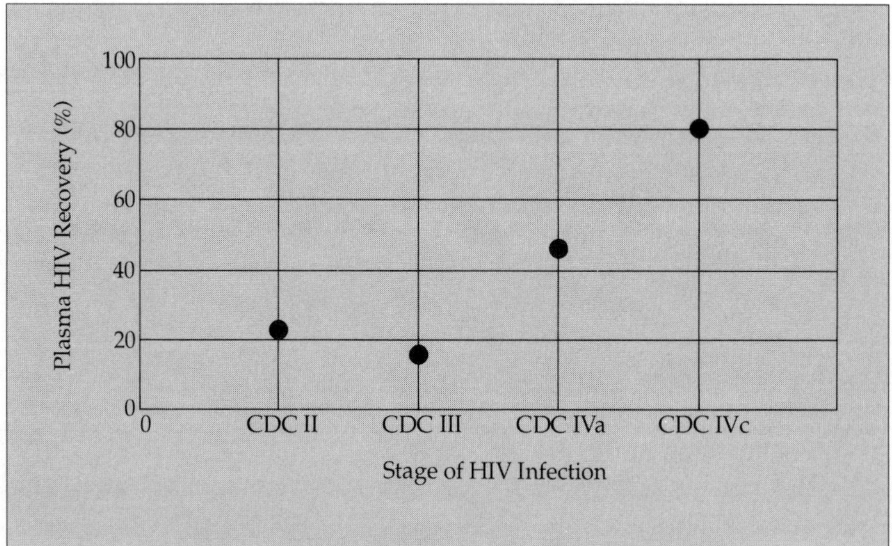

FIGURE 4. Recovery of plasma-associated HIV from patients with different stages of infection.
CDC group II: asymptomatic
CDC group III: persistent generalized lymphadenopathy
CDC group IVa: symptomatic (AIDS-related complex)
CDC group IVc: opportunistic infections (AIDS)

the Centers for Disease Control (CDC) recommends that any seropositive person be considered infectious. Representative isolation rates from various asymptomatic and symptomatic seropositive groups are shown in Table II.

Current HIV culture techniques have an undefined sensitivity; therefore, the reported isolation rates from different laboratories vary. At the University of Washington, we have developed a very sensitive HIV culture procedure that is providing new insight into the prevalence of HIV recovery from HIV-seropositive persons. We have shown greater than 98-percent recovery of HIV from the peripheral blood lymphocytes of 204 seropositive persons, irrespective of CDC group. (See "Clinical Manifestations and Approach to Management of HIV Infection and AIDS" on page 27 for a discussion of the CDC classification of HIV infection.) Our cross-sectional studies have demonstrated that HIV is more often isolated from the plasma of seropositive, symptomatic patients than from the plasma of asymptomatic patients (Figure 4). This suggests a higher HIV replicating load with more advanced disease. Prospective studies are under way to ascertain if the presence of plasma viremia in asymptomatic individuals is a harbinger of disease progression. We also have found that about 50 percent of neurologically asymptomatic, CDC group III (persistent generalized lymphadenopathy) homosexual men have both culture evidence—that is, positive cerebrospinal fluid cultures for HIV—and immunologic evidence for occult central nervous system infection with HIV. Prospective studies are in progress to determine the outcome of early central nervous system infection in this population.

Indications for HIV isolations: Present and future

Until HIV culture is standardized and of generally higher sensitivity, it must be considered a research supplement to the serologic diagnosis of HIV infection. There are, however, a number of potential applications for HIV culture in the clinical setting. First is the high-risk person with a suspected HIV infection (CDC group I) in whom a measurable antibody response has not occurred, either because the infection is acute or the person is unable to mount an immune response, as in the case of a congenital hypogammaglobulinemia, for example. (This also represents a potential application for viral antigen detection.) Secondly, the infant born to an HIV-seropositive mother may have maternal HIV IgG present for the first six to 15 months of life. Since HIV-IgM testing is not yet available, HIV culture and antigen detection are the only confirmatory tests for HIV infection in neonates. Third is HIV culture of cerebrospinal fluid from the seropositive patient with chronic central nervous system disease suggestive of AIDS dementia, or with any of several other neurologic syndromes where HIV is one of the potential etiologic candidates. HIV culture and the rapid detection of HIV infection also will become more clinically important when ef-

Table III Guidelines for HIV Antibody Testing

Decrease Transmission:
1. All blood and organ (including semen) donors
2. Persons who consider themselves at risk for HIV infection
3. Persons with a sexually transmitted disease
4. Intravenous drug abusers
5. Persons who received blood transfusions between 1978 and 1985
6. Women of childbearing age with identifiable risk for infection (including those planning surrogate motherhood)
7. Persons planning marriage where the seroprevalence is 0.1 percent or greater
8. Male and female prostitutes
9. Persons admitted to hospitals in those age groups deemed to have a high prevalence of HIV infection
10. Persons in correctional institutions (and perhaps institutions for chronic psychiatric care where regulation of sexual activity may be difficult and segregation may be necessary to protect seronegative persons)

Diagnosis:
1. Generalized lymphadenopathy
2. Unexplained dementia or encephalopathy
3. Chronic unexplained fever
4. Chronic unexplained diarrhea
5. Unexplained weight loss or wasting syndrome
6. Tuberculosis
7. Chronic candidiasis
8. Kaposi's sarcoma
9. Primary lymphoma of the brain
10. Generalized herpes virus infection affecting a patient greater than one month old
11. (Aseptic meningitis)*
12. (Unexplained interstitial pneumonia)
13. (Idiopathic thrombocytopenic purpura)
14. (Heterophile negative infectious mononucleosis)*
15. (Unexplained psychosis or peripheral neuropathy)
16. (Any person with either a definitively or presumptively diagnosed opportunistic infection, malignancy or other disease consistent with AIDS)
17. (Any infant born to a high-risk mother)†
18. For patients less than 13 years old:
    —Unexplained recurrent bacterial infections
    —Lymphoid interstitial pneumonia/pulmonary lymphoid hyperplasia
    —(Unexplained failure to thrive)
    —(Unexplained developmental delay)
    —(Unexplained parotitis)
    —(Unexplained hepatitis)
    —(Unexplained cardiomyopathy)

After *Morbid Mortal Weekly Rep* 1987; 36(31):509-515 and *Morbid Mortal Weekly Rep* 1987; 36(1S):3S-15S.

Parenthetical additions represent our own recommendations.

*Caveat: For the initially HIV seronegative person, serologic testing should be repeated at six weeks, and if still negative, then again at three and six months to exclude an early infection.

†The presence of anti-HIV IgG, by itself, is insufficient evidence for HIV infection because passively acquired maternal antibodies may persist for up to 15 months after birth (*Morbid Mortal Weekly Rep* 1987; 36:225-230).

fective antiviral chemotherapy becomes available.

Clinical utility of HIV tests

It is easy to see how a variety of HIV diagnostic tests can be used clinically. For example, a patient may report fatigue and weight loss to a physician. After taking a medical history, the physician determines that the patient is a member of a high-risk group for HIV infection. Following consent, the patient's serum is tested by enzyme immunoassay for detection of antibody to HIV. If the serum is repeatedly reactive by enzyme immunoassay, it is then tested by Western blot to confirm the presence of specific antibody to HIV viral proteins. If positive, the patient is then counseled and followed for changes in clinical status. In the future, it is likely that such patients may be tested for specific antibody to the core protein p24 using second-generation assays, or for the presence of the p24 core antigen. If there is a lower titer of antibody to p24 or if antigen is present in serum, the patient may need closer monitoring for disease progression. A patient treated with anti-HIV chemotherapy may be monitored for drug efficacy by viral culture or by assays for the presence of viral antigen or viral nucleic acid.

Guidelines for HIV antibody testing

Establishing the laboratory confirmation of HIV infection has two important functions: to establish a diagnosis and to interrupt transmission of the virus. Serologic testing, combined with counseling, can modify behavior and encourage low-risk sexual practices, particularly among some homosexual men.

To assist the clinician in deciding who would most benefit from serologic testing, we have outlined the current U.S. Public Health Service guidelines for HIV antibody testing (Table III). These guidelines may be subdivided into those recommendations that directly assist with decreasing HIV transmission and those that help the clinician to diagnose HIV infection. In certain instances we have made suggestions to increase the scope of testing; these suggestions should prompt the clinician to search for a history of high-risk group membership and to obtain consent for HIV antibody testing. For early HIV infection (which could present as either an acute mononucleosis-like syndrome or acute aseptic meningitis), repeated serologic testing at six, nine and 24 weeks may be necessary because of the delayed antibody response to HIV infection.

Although AIDS remains, for the most part, a clinical diagnosis, it is unusual under current clinical practice for a diagnosis to be confirmed without prior HIV serology. However, in the absence of certain definitively diagnosed indicator diseases required by the current case definition (*Morbid Mortal Weekly Rep* 1987; 36(1S):3S-14S), a positive serologic test for HIV antibody is required to confirm a diagnosis of AIDS in the following instances:

A) Definitively diagnosed disseminated coccidioidomycosis or histoplasmosis; isosporiasis; recurrent *Salmonella* septicemia; extrapulmonary tuberculosis; disseminated mycobacterial disease caused by mycobacteria other than *M. tuberculosis*; non-Hodgkin's lymphoma of high-grade pathologic type and of B-cell or unknown immunologic phenotype; Kaposi's sarcoma or primary lymphoma of the brain affecting patients who are 60 years old or older; dementia/encephalopathy; wasting syndrome; patients with syndromes indicative of AIDS but who have received immunosuppressive/cytotoxic therapy within the three months prior to developing an indicator disease or who develop certain lymphoreticular malignancies within the three-month period after developing an indicator disease; and patients with a genetic immunodeficiency syndrome or an acquired immunodeficiency syndrome atypical of HIV infection, such as hypogammaglobulinemia.

B) Presumptively diagnosed esophageal candidiasis, cytomegalovirus retinitis, *Pneumocystis carinii* pneumonia, Kaposi's sarcoma, toxoplasmosis of the brain affecting patients older than one month, and lymphoid interstitial pneumonia/pulmonary lymphoid hyperplasia in children less than 13 years old.

Summary

Persons with HIV infection develop antibodies to several HIV-encoded proteins. The enzyme immunoassay currently used for screening blood donations and patient specimens detects antibody to multiple viral antigens, and demonstrates greater than 99-percent sensitivity and specificity. In populations having a high prevalence of infection (for example, 66 percent), the predictive value of a repeatably positive enzyme immunoassay is greater than 99 percent. However, in populations where the prevalence of infection is low (for example, less than 1 percent), such as blood donors, the predictive value of a repeatably positive enzyme immunoassay is only about 60 percent. Other, more specific methods—such as Western blot, immunofluorescence assay, or radioimmunoprecipitation—are used to confirm the presence of antibody to individual viral proteins in serum specimens that are repeatably positive by enzyme immunoassay.

Second-generation tests for antibody to individual, specific viral proteins encoded by *env* and *gag* genes use either recombinant proteins produced in bacteria or chemically synthesized peptides. These tests are more specific than current enzyme immunoassays and are cheaper and safer to produce. Additionally, detection of antibodies to individual proteins may be important in monitoring disease progression.

Third-generation assays have been developed to detect viral antigen or viral RNA and DNA. Detection of viral antigen may be important early in infection, late in disease, and during antiviral chemotherapy. Viral culture also may be used to evaluate efficacy of therapy and vaccination.

Future development of laboratory tests for HIV detection must take into account the recent isolation and characterization of HIV-2, HTLV-IV and other HIV types from Africa. Because HIV-1 and HIV-2 exhibit antigenic cross-reactivity only between *gag* and *pol* proteins and not *env* proteins, blood infected with HIV-2 may not be detected by current enzyme immunoassay screens that are based on detection of HIV-1 antibodies.

Additional Reading

Allain, J-P, Paul, D.A., Senn, D. and Laurian, Y. 1986. Serological Markers in Early Stages of Human Immunodeficiency Virus Infection in Haemophiliacs. *Lancet* 8518:1233-1236.

Barre-Sinoussi, F., Chermann, J-C, Rey, F., Nugeryre, M.T. *et al.* 1983. Isolation of a T-lymphotropic retrovirus from a patient at risk for acquired immune deficiency syndrome (AIDS). *Science* 220:868-871.

Chang, N.T., Huang, J., Ghrayeb, J., McKinney, S., Chanda, P.K., Chang, T.W., Putney, S., Sarngadharan, M.G., Wong-Staal, F. and Gallo, R.C. 1985. An HTLV-III Peptide Produced by Recombinant DNA is Immunoreactive with Sera from Patients with AIDS. *Nature* 315:151-154.

Gallo, R.C., Sarin, P.S., Geimann, E.P., Robert-Guroff, M., Richardson, E. *et al.* 1983. Isolation of human T-cell leukemia virus in acquired immune deficiency syndrome (AIDS). *Science* 220:865-867.

Gallo, D., Diggs, J.L., Shell, G.R., Dailey, P.J., Hoffman, M.N. and Riggs, J.L. 1986. Comparison of Detection of Antibody to the Acquired Immune Deficiency Syndrome Virus by Enzyme Immunoassay, Immunofluorescence, and Western Blot Methods. *J Clin Micro* 23:1049-1051.

McDougal, J.S., Cort, S.P., Kennedy, M.S., Cabridilla, C.D., Feorino, P.M., Francis, D.P., Hicks, D., Kalyanaraman, V.S. and Martin, L.S. 1985. Immunoassay for the Detection and Quantitation of Infectious Human Retrovirus, Lymphadenopathy-Associated Virus (LAV). *J Immunological Methods* 76:171-183.

Sarngadharan, M.G., Popovic, M., Bruch, L., Schupbach, J. and Gallo, R.C. 1984. Antibodies Reactive with Human T-Lymphotropic Retroviruses (HTLV-III) in the Serum of Patients with AIDS. *Science* 224:506-508.

Clinical Manifestations and Approach to Management of HIV Infection and AIDS

by Ann C. Collier, M.D., Terence C. Gayle, M.D., and Fredrick H. Bahls, M.D., Ph.D.

Persons with human immunodeficiency virus (HIV) infection show a broad spectrum of clinical presentations that range from asymptomatic to life-threatening. Conceptually, clinical issues involve those that relate to HIV infection and those that are complications of HIV-induced immunodeficiency. The number and variety of specific infectious and malignant complications associated with acquired immunodeficiency syndrome (AIDS) continue to expand, but so has information about diagnosis and treatment. Many complications of AIDS are treatable, and treatment may prolong survival and improve the quality of life for affected persons. However, therapy for some complications is suboptimal. Some widely used treatments are experimental, and for other complications, no specific treatment is available. Multiple opportunistic complications frequently coexist and some require lifelong treatment. However, the principles of care are no different for this problem than for other medical conditions.

Classification of HIV infection

The Centers for Disease Control introduced the classification scheme that is most widely used to characterize the spectrum of disorders caused by HIV. Persons infected with HIV are grouped into four main categories (Table I). Since the natural history of HIV is incompletely understood, this scheme was not designed to have prognostic significance. Persons are classified into the highest group for which they meet the assignment criteria.

Group I includes acute HIV infection, which usually occurs one to twelve weeks following exposure. This event may be asymptomatic; may resemble mononucleosis with malaise, fever, lymphadenopathy, rash, headache and/or myalgias/arthralgias; or may result in aseptic meningitis. The symptoms are usually self-limited, and treatment is supportive. Diagnosis of Group I infection requires documentation of HIV antibody seroconversion.

Asymptomatic HIV-seropositive individuals comprise Group II. Group III HIV disease includes persons with persistent generalized lymphadenopathy, which is defined by the presence of lymph nodes measuring at least 1 centimeter in diameter in at least two extrainguinal areas for at least three months. Many persons with persistent generalized lymphadenopathy are asymptomatic, although some have mild constitutional symptoms such as night sweats or fatigue. Group II or III patients may have laboratory abnormalities such as leukopenia, lymphopenia, thrombocytopenia, hypergammaglobulinemia and/or anemia. Patients with Group II or III infection also appear to have equal risk for the subsequent development of overt AIDS.

Group IV disease, which includes AIDS and AIDS-related complex (ARC), is divided into five subgroups (Table I). Subgroup A includes persons with constitutional symptoms, such as persistent unexplained fever, significant weight loss and/or diarrhea without identifiable cause. This syndrome was known previously as ARC. Although the term ARC has been widely used to refer to constitutional symptoms and a wasting syndrome associated with HIV, no uniform definition has been established. Before attributing symptoms to HIV infection, other potential etiologies must be excluded. Directed laboratory studies should be based on the patient's symptoms and signs. Even in the absence of identifiable complications, ARC may cause extreme debilitation. Current approaches to treatment include nutritional support, treatment with zidovudine (formerly known as azidothymidine or AZT) for patients with severely depressed T4 helper cells, specific treatment of any complicating infections, and psychosocial support. Zidovudine clearly has been shown to benefit patients with previous *Pneumocystis carinii* pneumonia or severe ARC.

Persons with significant neurologic disease fall into subgroup B of Group IV, unless they also have a specific opportunistic disease characteristic of AIDS. Group IV, subgroup C is itself divided into two categories: C-1 includes persons with one or more of the 12 opportunistic infections included in the 1985 Centers for Disease Control surveillance definition of AIDS. C-2 refers to six other infectious diseases, including recurrent *Salmonella* bacteremia and multidermatomal herpes zoster. Subgroup D refers to the malignancies recognized in the present Centers for Disease Control surveillance definition, including Kaposi's sarcoma and non-Hodgkins lymphoma. Subgroup E includes a variety of other severe conditions.

The signs, symptoms and associated complications of HIV infection in children are somewhat different from those in adults. The Centers for Disease Control classification scheme for the manifestations of

Dr. Collier is a University of Washington assistant professor of medicine and is director of the AIDS Clinic at Harborview Medical Center. Dr. Gayle is a UW acting instructor of psychiatry and behavioral sciences and is a Veterans Administration Fellow in the UW Robert Wood Johnson Clinical Scholar Program. Dr. Bahls is an acting instructor of neurology and a senior fellow in physiology at the UW and is an attending neurologist at the Seattle VA Medical Center.

Table I Centers for Disease Control (CDC) Classification System for HIV Infection

Group		Description
1		Acute HIV infection, requiring documentation of seroconversion
2		Asymptomatic seropositives; no current or previous signs or symptoms of infection
3		Persistent generalized lymphadenopathy; palpable lymphadenopathy at 2 or more extrainguinal sites
4		Severe AIDS-related diseases
	A	Constitutional disease; unexplained fever or diarrhea for more than 1 month or loss of more than 10 percent of body weight
	B	Neurologic disease; unexplained dementia, myelopathy or neuropathy
	C-1	Opportunistic infection; symptomatic or invasive disease due to 1 of the 12 secondary infectious diseases specified in original CDC surveillance definition for AIDS*
	C-2	Other infections; symptomatic or invasive disease due to 1 of 6 other specified infectious diseases: oral hairy leukoplakia, multidermatomal herpes zoster, recurrent *Salmonella* bacteremia, nocardiosis, tuberculosis, or oral candidiasis
	D	Opportunistic malignancies of CDC surveillance definition: Kaposi's sarcoma, non-Hodgkin's lymphoma, primary central nervous system lymphoma
	E	Other conditions

Pneumocystis carinii pneumonia, chronic cryptosporidiosis, toxoplasmosis, extraintestinal strongyloidiasis, isosporiasis, candidiasis (esophageal, bronchial or pulmonary), cryptococcosis, histoplasmosis, mycobacterial infection with *Mycobacterium avium* complex or *M. kansasii*, cytomegalovirus infection, chronic mucocutaneous or disseminated herpes simplex virus infection, progressive multifocal leukoencephalopathy pediatric AIDS is described in Table II and in the "Additional Reading" list at the end of this article.

Systemic infections

The most common infection in patients with HIV infection, oral candidiasis, frequently precedes other opportunistic infections (Figure 1). Treatment with oral nystatin or topical clotrimazole troches is generally effective, but continued suppressive therapy is usually necessary. Ketoconazole is useful where these regimens are not effective. In addition to ameliorating symptoms, treatment may prevent symptomatic esophogeal involvement. For patients suspected to have esophagitis, it is important to eliminate other diagnostic possibilities such as herpes simplex virus or cytomegalovirus. Invasive candidiasis may occur in AIDS patients but is far less common than in other immunocompromised hosts.

Pneumocystis carinii pneumonia (PCP) is the most common serious infection that occurs with AIDS. *P. carinii* is a widely distributed protozoan to which most healthy persons are exposed in childhood. PCP is a typical example of opportunistic infections that occur with AIDS; reactivation of latent colonization puts immunocompromised hosts at risk for severe pulmonary infection. Symptoms of fever, malaise, non-productive cough, and dyspnea may gradually progress over days to weeks, although fulminant respiratory failure also may occur. Chest radiographs typically show diffuse, bilateral, interstitial infiltrates, but findings may be subtle and X-rays occasionally may be normal. Because cultures and serologic tests currently are not clinically useful, diagnosis of PCP requires demonstration of organisms in induced sputum, fluid from nasotrachial suction or bronchial-alveolar lavage, or transbronchial biopsy.

Reported mortality for PCP is 10 to 30 percent, but may be as high as 85 percent if the pneumonia is severe enough to require ventilatory support. PCP is treated with trimethoprim-sulfamethoxazole, pentamidine or dapsone-trimethoprim for 21 days (Table III). These regimens are equally effective, although side effects are common. More than 50 percent of patients are unable to tolerate a full course of the initial two therapies, and require a switch from one regimen to another. Trimethoprim-sulfamethoxazole has been associated with drug-induced fever, rash, leukopenia and elevated transaminases. Pentamidine may cause hypotension, hypoglycemia, hyperglycemia, renal insufficiency, leukopenia, and elevations in liver function tests. It should be given by slow (>1 hour) intravenous infusion to avoid the sterile abscesses it commonly causes if administered intramuscularly. In most situations, therapy should be initiated parenterally. If patients respond well or are extremely stable at diagnosis, oral treatment can be considered. Alternative therapies are under investigation. In addition to antimicrobial therapy, supportive therapy is crucial.

Chemoprophylaxis for PCP in AIDS is controversial; regimens that have been used include trimethoprim-sulfamethoxazole two to seven days per week, dapsone, intramuscular or inhaled pentamidine, and weekly Fansidar™. Although data clearly supports

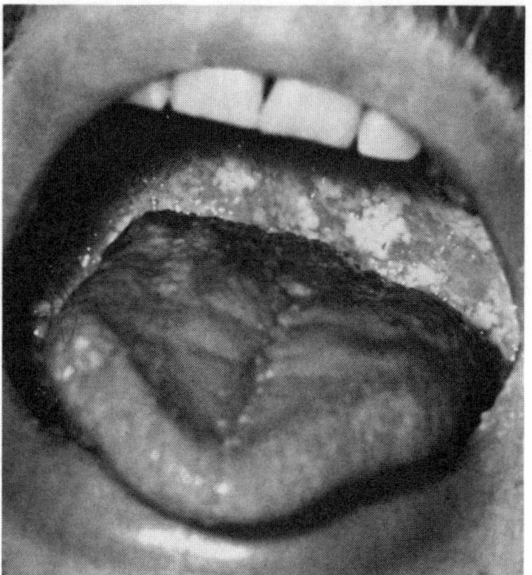

FIGURE 1. Oral candidiasis, showing characteristic adherent white plaques and erythematous mucosa.

the use of prophylaxis for PCP in immunosuppressed children, similar data is not currently available for AIDS patients. Zidovudine has been shown to decrease the occurrence of opportunistic infections in patients who have had one episode of PCP, but the long-term safety of treatment in conjunction with specific therapy to prevent PCP is unknown. The apparent lack of systemic absorption and side effects of inhaled pentamidine (30-150 mg biweekly by nebulizer that delivers 0.5-2.5 micron particles) has created significant interest in this agent as a means of PCP prophylaxis.

The pathogenicity of the atypical mycobacteria, *Mycobacterium avium-intracellulare* (MAI), in persons with AIDS is controversial, although its high prevalence is not disputed. More than half of patients dying with AIDS have disseminated MAI at autopsy. Symptoms attributed to it include fever, malaise, weight loss, malabsorption and diarrhea. Blood cultures are the most useful diagnostic test for detection. This organism often is highly resistant to conventional antituberculous therapy. Although a variety of drug combinations have been used for MAI treatment, their utility has not yet been demonstrated. If treatment is undertaken, multiple agents should be used.

Infection with *Mycobacterium tuberculosis* also occurs in persons with HIV infection. All HIV-seropositive persons should have skin testing for evidence of exposure to *M. tuberculosis*. Tuberculosis may be the first opportunistic infection to occur in some HIV-infected persons. The guidelines for tuberculosis treatment in patients with HIV or AIDS are fairly similar to those for other patients. The response to therapy is usually good.

A number of viral infections are associated with AIDS, including several members of the herpes family. Reactivation of varicella zoster virus in HIV-seropositive persons suggests immunologic impairment and may precede more serious conditions. Herpes simplex virus may cause persistent ulcerations in the genital or perirectal area in patients with AIDS or HIV infection. Acyclovir is an effective antiviral treatment for varicella zoster virus in compromised hosts, and for therapy and prophylaxis of herpes simplex virus.

Table II Centers for Disease Control Classification System for HIV Infection in Children Under 13 Years of Age

Class	Infection
P-0	Indeterminate infection
P-1	Asymptomatic infection
	A. Normal immune function
	B. Abnormal immune function
	C. Immune function not tested
P-2	Symptomatic infection
	A. Non-specific findings
	B. Progressive neurologic disease
	C. Lymphoid interstitial pneumonitis
	D. Secondary infectious diseases
	D-1 Specified in adult surveillance definition
	D-2 Recurrent serious bacterial infection (two or more within two years)
	D-3 Other specified infections*
	E. Secondary cancers
	E-1 Specified in adult surveillance definition
	E-2 Cancers possibly secondary to HIV
	F. Other diseases; children with other conditions possibly associated with HIV, such as cardiopathy, thrombocytopenia or dermatitis

*Oral candidiasis for two months or more
Two or more episodes of herpes stomatitis within one year
Multidermatomal or disseminated herpes zoster

Of the viral infections commonly associated with AIDS, cytomegalovirus causes the most devastating clinical problem. Asymptomatic infection is common, but the virus frequently disseminates and causes retinitis that can lead to blindness. Cytomegalovirus retinitis is characterized by progressive retinal inflammation with hemorrhages and exudates. Clinical deterioration can occur over days to weeks. Uncontrolled studies with the experimental drug ganciclovir, also known as DHPG (dihydroxy-propyl-methyl-guanine), suggest stabilization of vision in two-thirds of those treated. Maintenance therapy is necessary to prevent relapse and is given intravenously five to seven times a week.

Opportunistic malignancies

The most common malignant disease associated with AIDS is Kaposi's sarcoma, which is far more common among homosexual men than among heterosexuals with AIDS. Its cause is not known. Cutaneous involvement is almost universal in Kaposi's sarcoma (Figure 2). Gastrointestinal involvement, including the mouth, is common. Kaposi's sarcoma lesions may be erythematous, violaceous, black or multicolored. Yellow halos around lesions are common. Lesions may be macular, papular or nodular, and usually are asymptomatic. Since early lesions may be difficult to distinguish from traumatic bruises, careful observation of suspected lesions may be indicated for a few weeks before biopsy. Therapeutic approaches include observation for limited cutaneous disease, single or multi-agent chemotherapy, alpha interferon and/or local irradiation. Persons rarely die of Kaposi's sarcoma itself but are likely to eventually develop other opportunistic infections.

Neurologic complications

Although AIDS was recognized as a clinical entity in 1981, the extent and variety of neurologic involvement was not appreciated immediately. Clinical involve-

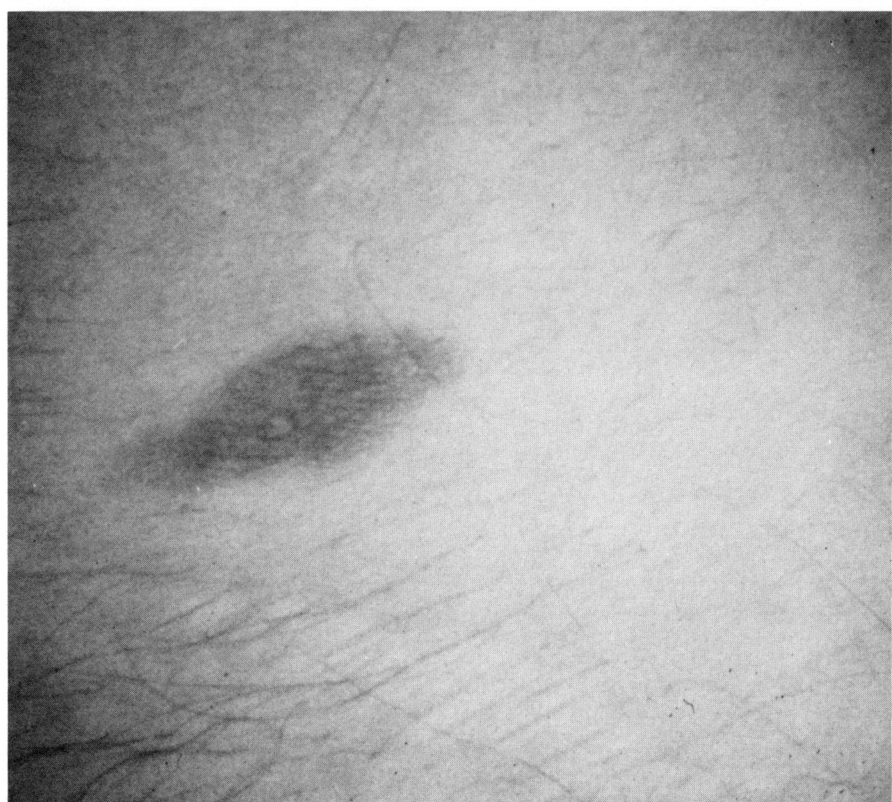

FIGURE 2. Cutaneous Kaposi's sarcoma, showing an early lesion of a non-tender, solitary, erythematous macule.

ment of the nervous system occurs in at least 40 percent of AIDS patients and may be the initial manifestation of HIV infection in 10 to 30 percent of patients. Several neuropathological studies of AIDS patients have found evidence of central nervous system disease in as many as 90 percent of cases. The discrepancy between clinical and pathological estimates of central nervous system involvement is probably due to the presence of subclinical nervous system disease and to the failure to recognize subtle signs of nervous system involvement in patients with devastating systemic disease.

HIV infection can result in a broad spectrum of neurologic disease. No currently recognized characteristics of patients with HIV infection predict the subsequent occurrence of neurologic disease or its nature. We will discuss the most common types of neurologic presentations associated with HIV infection and emphasize those conditions for which specific therapy is available.

AIDS dementia complex

The most common neurologic presentation of patients with HIV infection is progressive dementia, which has been called the AIDS dementia complex or HIV-associated encephalopathy and was previously referred to as subacute encephalitis or subacute encephalopathy. While this syndrome occurs most commonly after diagnosis of overt AIDS, it also may be the first sign of HIV infection. The onset of symptoms is usually insidious but occasionally they may present with a fulminant course over a few days. This syndrome carries a grave prognosis with a mean survival of approximately four months. Early signs and symptoms in

patients with this syndrome can be extremely subtle (Table IV). In the later stages, patients become demented and the majority have other neurological signs. The most common finding on computerized tomography is cortical atrophy. Cerebrospinal fluid studies commonly reveal a mild to moderate increase in protein and sometimes a mild mononuclear pleocytosis. On neuropathologic examination, the abnormalities are predominantly in the white matter and subcortical structures with sparing of the cerebral cortex. Diffuse pallor of the white matter is the most characteristic finding, with clusters of foamy macrophages and multinucleated giant cells present in severe cases.

While the precise etiology of this syndrome is not yet known, isolation of HIV from brains of affected patients and the demonstration of antibodies to HIV in cerebrospinal fluid suggest that the AIDS dementia complex is due to direct infection of the brain by HIV. HIV appears to primarily infect microglia and macrophages rather than neurons or astroglia. No specific treatment for this syndrome has been found, although anecdotal reports suggest that zidovudine may benefit some patients. It is important to emphasize that patients with other, more treatable causes of central nervous system involvement may present in precisely the same manner (see below), and that the diagnosis of the AIDS dementia complex remains one of exclusion.

Mass lesions

Another common neurologic presentation of patients with HIV infection is with an intracerebral mass lesion. Such patients may have headache, focal or generalized

---

Table III Treatment Regimens for *Pneumocystis carinii* Pneumonia

Accepted Alternatives:*

Trimethoprim-sulfamethoxazole

—(20 mg/kg/day of trimethoprim and 100 mg/kg/day of sulfamethoxazole, given q 6 h; intravenous or oral)

Pentamidine

—(4 mg/kg/day, given intravenously by slow infusion >1 hr/dose)

Dapsone and Trimethoprim

—(dapsone 100 mg/day; oral)

—(trimethoprim 20 mg/kg/day given q 6 h; oral)

Investigational Treatments:

Inhaled pentamidine

Dimethyl fluoro-ornithine (DMFO)

Trimetrexate

*21-day therapy recommended; no benefit for dual regimens (see text)

Table IV Signs and Symptoms of AIDS Dementia Complex

Cognitive (66%)	Motor (45%)	Behavioral (39%)	Other (20%)
Early:			
Forgetfulness	Decreased balance	Apathy	Headache
Decreased concentration	Lower extremity weakness	Social withdrawal	Seizure
Confusion	Handwriting changes		
Late:			
Dementia	Psychomotor retardation	Indifferent	Organic psychosis
Confusion	Ataxia	Awake	Tremor
Memory loss	Increased tone	Wide-eyed stare	Frontal release signs
	Weakness	Incontinence	

Adapted from Navia *et al.* 1986.

seizures, focal weakness or encephalopathy. On examination, patients may have papilledema, hemiparesis, hemisensory loss, aphasia and/or mental status abnormalities. Computed tomography (CT) and/or magnetic resonance (MR) scanning can determine the presence of a mass lesion in such patients (Figure 3). However, the exact cause of a mass lesion in a given patient can be determined only by brain biopsy, since no particular etiologic agent has either a pathognomonic clinical presentation or neuroradiologic appearance. Similarly, while lumbar puncture should be performed in all patients in whom CT or MR scanning does not show significant mass effect, cerebrospinal fluid studies often are not specific for a given cause.

The most common cause of central nervous system mass lesions in patients with HIV infection is toxoplasmosis (Figure 4). It is reasonable in most cases to begin empiric treatment with sulfadiazine and pyrimethamine. Patients with toxoplasmosis infection generally show both clinical and radiologic improvement one to two weeks after therapy begins. Therapy in patients who improve needs to be maintained lifelong unless side effects develop. Those patients who are unable to tolerate sulfadiazine may respond to clindamycin therapy, although there is little data on its efficacy.

Patients with mass lesions in the central nervous system who fail to respond to empiric therapy for toxoplasmosis should be considered for brain biopsy if the lesion is accessible. An MR scan may reveal additional, more accessible lesions in those patients whose CT scans reveal only a deep lesion. Primary central nervous system lymphoma is the second most common cause of mass lesions in AIDS patients. A common presenting feature is cranial polyneuropathy. Diagnosis is made by biopsy or, more commonly, on postmortem examination. Since the diagnosis often is made postmortem, there is little information on the best therapy. A few patients have shown some response to whole brain irradiation.

Other, less common causes of mass lesions in patients with AIDS include atypical mycobacteria, tuberculosis, cryptococcus, candida, and progressive multifocal leukoencephalopathy. It is not uncommon for patients to have multiple central nervous system complications, and new diagnoses should be considered if new symptoms appear.

Meningitis

Meningitis is another neurologic presentation of patients with HIV infection. *Cryptococcus neoformans* is its most frequent infectious cause. Symptoms may include fever, headache, encephalopathy or seizures. Patients often have no meningismis. Diagnosis is made by finding elevated cryptococcal antigen in the cerebrospinal fluid. Cryptococcal meningitis is treated with amphotericin B and with 5-flucytosine, if tolerated. Like patients with toxoplasmosis, patients with cryptococcal

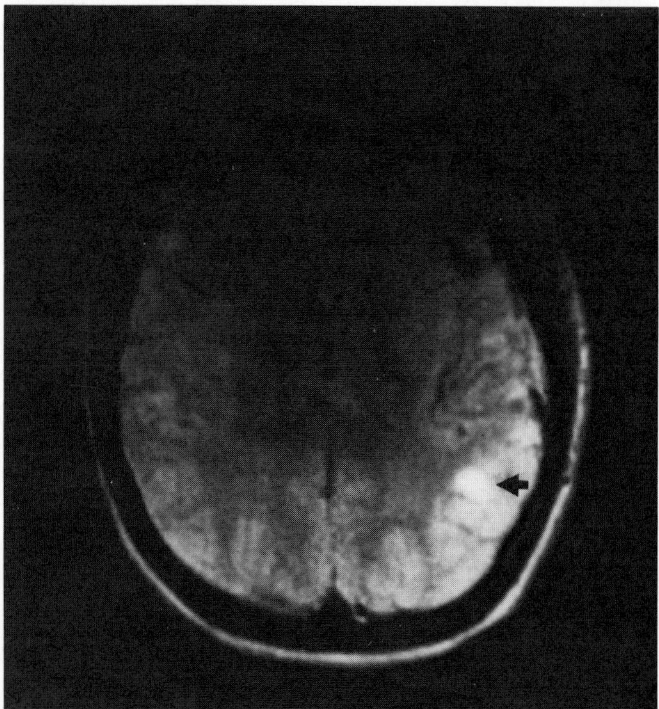

FIGURE 3A. Magnetic resonance image of the brain of a patient with progressive ataxia, paresthesias and mental status changes. This cut shows one of multiple lesions present.

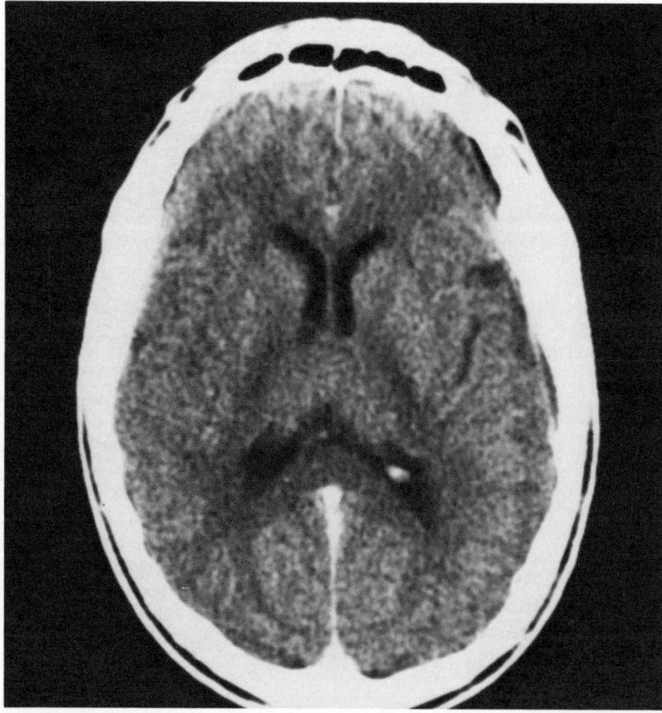

FIGURE 3B. The patient's computed tomography scan at the same time was normal. The lesion was visible on a repeat CT performed one month later. This case demonstrates that MR may detect lesions not apparent on CT.

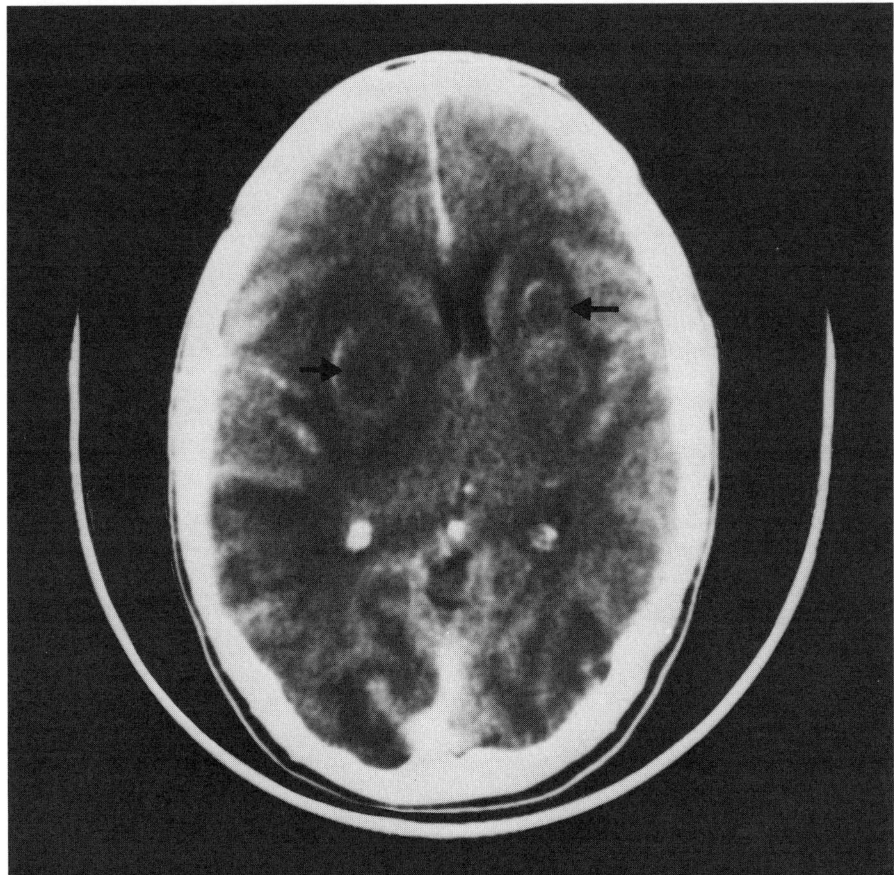

FIGURE 4. This patient presented with focal motor seizures and left-sided weakness. Computed tomography (CT) revealed multiple, enhancing mass lesions which, on postmortem, were shown to be abscesses caused by toxoplasmosis. Other causes of central nervous system mass lesions may have an identical appearance on CT scan.

infection need chronic therapy to prevent relapse.

Atypical aseptic meningitis is another type of meningitis seen in patients with HIV infection. It typically occurs in patients who have no other manifestations of HIV infection. Patients may have headache, fever, meningeal signs, cranial nerve involvement (usually the 5th, 7th and 8th cranial nerves) and long tract signs such as hyperreflexia. Examination of cerebrospinal fluid reveals a mononuclear pleocytosis and increased opening pressure. The cause of this syndrome is unknown, although HIV itself is suspected. In most patients, the illness is self-limited.

Spinal cord syndromes

Several types of spinal cord involvement are associated with HIV infection, the most common of which is vacuolar myelopathy. Patients develop progressive paraparesis, spasticity, ataxia, incontinence and extensor plantar responses. Patients frequently also have the AIDS dementia complex. Myelography and cerebrospinal fluid examination are normal. Pathologically, white matter vacuolation and demyelination are present most prominently in the dorsal and lateral (corticospinal tract) columns. The etiology is unknown, but the frequent association with AIDS dementia complex suggests direct infection of the spinal cord with HIV.

Another type of spinal cord involvement is transverse or ascending myelitis. These patients have back pain, usually in the thoracic region; flaccid paresis below the level of the lesion; a sensory level; hyporeflexia and a neurogenic bladder. They may progress to quadraparesis with cranial nerve involvement. Myelography is normal. Cerebrospinal fluid may be normal or a lymphocytic pleocytosis may occur. Both cytomegalovirus and herpes simplex type 2 have been recovered from the spinal cords of such patients. Since cord compression from epidural abscess or metastatic tumor also can occur in patients with HIV infection, myelography is mandatory in all patients who show evidence of spinal cord involvement.

Peripheral neuropathy

Two distinct syndromes of peripheral nerve involvement have been reported in patients with HIV infection. A chronic inflammatory polyneuropathy may occur, most commonly in patients without other manifestations of HIV infection. It may present in a variety of forms, including mononeuritis multiplex, distal symmetrical or asymmetrical polyneuropathy, or with a Guillain-Barre syndrome. All patients typically have fever and malaise. Cerebrospinal fluid IgG index is increased and nerve biopsy shows inflammatory changes. The course is usually benign with spontaneous remission. Plasmapheresis may be of benefit in cases with a prolonged course.

In patients with overt AIDS, a distal symmetric polyneuropathy is the most common peripheral neuropathy. These patients have painful dysesthesias that may be incapacitating and symmetric sensory loss that only rarely includes motor involvement. Diagnostic studies usually are unrevealing and no clear etiology has been determined. Diphenylhydantoin, carbamazepine or one of the tricyclic antidepressants may benefit patients with severe neuropathic pain.

Neurologic summary

HIV infection should be considered in any patient with an unusual neurologic disorder. Such patients should undergo evaluation that includes neuroradiologic examination (CT and/or MR), cerebrospinal fluid examination, and myelography or brain biopsy in certain cases. It is important to recognize that patients often may have more than one type of neurologic involvement and require frequent reassessment.

Neuropsychiatric manifestations of HIV infection

There is growing recognition of the wide variety of organic mental disorders associated with HIV and AIDS. These neuropsychiatric disorders range from subtle personality changes to severe dementia. Delirium is the most frequent acute organic mental disorder seen in AIDS patients. It begins abruptly (usually hours to days) and is characterized by clouded consciousness and disorientation that fluctuate over the course of a day. Delirium also is associated with incoherent speech, altered sleep-wake pattern, perceptual disturbances such as hallucinations, and increased or decreased psychomotor activity. In AIDS patients, delirium most often is due to underlying systemic or central nervous system diseases and frequently to drug toxicity. Because the underlying conditions are often treatable, it is important to conduct a thorough medical evaluation of any patient with an emerging delirium.

The AIDS dementia complex (described above) is the chronic organic mental disorder seen most often in patients with HIV infection. Because cognitive dysfunction can frighten patients, it is important not to overlook the early, subtle symptoms of dementia nor to attribute them solely to the emotional reaction to a diagnosis of HIV infection or AIDS. About one-third of patients display increasing apathy and social withdrawal that may mimic major depression. These "negative" symptoms often do not respond to standard antidepressant medications. Other symptoms that should lead to suspicion of early dementia include sleep changes (particularly hypersomnia), impaired judgment, avoidance of complex tasks, increased reliance on lists, obsessive rumination, and increased sensitivity to alcohol and prescribed medications. It is not unusual to see presentations of dementia with an overlying (and reversible) delirium.

As many as 80 percent of AIDS patients without documented neurologic complications show subclinical cognitive impairment in formal neuropsychological testing. Preliminary research suggests that cognitive dysfunction may occur in a subset of patients with early stages of HIV infection. Because cognitive difficulties may be overlooked by a cursory mental status exam that relies upon orientation questions only, it is crucial that patients with HIV undergo initial assessment with a more thorough exam.

The Mini-Mental State Exam (Table V) is useful and can be administered at the bedside or in the office in 10 to 15 minutes. The initial mental status can serve as a baseline for comparison with subsequent exams. The exam by itself does not comprehensively evaluate cognitive function or dementia, but serves as a screening test for more gross dysfunction. (For example, patients may legitimately complain of memory problems, yet still score in the normal range of 24 or above.) For valid exam results, persons being tested must have greater than an eighth-grade education and not have significant sensory or motor deficits—such as impaired vision (for example, cytomegalovirus retinitis) or upper arm weakness—that might interfere with completion of some test questions. When patients show atypical psychiatric features and an organic mental disorder is suspected, it may be helpful to undertake formal neuropsychological testing.

Such testing is also very helpful in detecting milder cognitive impairment associated with central nervous system infection with HIV. This limited impairment may not constitute global dementia but may interfere with a patient's ability to perform more complex work tasks. With the recent addition of dementia associated with HIV infection to the Centers for Disease Control surveillance definition for AIDS, neuropsychological testing may become increasingly important to document cognitive impairment. Neurological evaluation as outlined in the previous section also is indicated. If the dementia is more severe, patients should be referred to an occupational therapist for an evaluation of daily activities (for example, telephoning, cooking, and taking medications) to determine the level of practical assistance needed.

As dementia progresses, psychotic features including hallucinations, delusions and agitated behavior may appear. These are best treated with low-dose, high-potency neuroleptics such as haloperidol or thiothixene. Other psychotropic medications—such as long-acting benzodiazepines (diazepam or chlordiazepoxide) and the more anticholinergic neuroleptics (chlorpromazine) — may actually worsen behavior and contribute to delirium. Management strategies may include schemes to help people remember appointments and medication schedules or reality orientation aids such as calendars, clocks and familiar attendants.

Psychiatrists have noted certain atypical psychiatric presentations in AIDS and ARC patients. These include organic mood syndromes (depression and mania) and atypical psychoses. These psychiatric syndromes can develop rapidly in individuals who have neither premorbid psychiatric history nor family history of

psychiatric disorders. HIV has been implicated as a probable etiologic factor, although other systemic and central nervous system diseases can produce these conditions.

True major depression usually responds to antidepressant medications. As has been observed in major depression associated with cancer, some but not all AIDS patients with major depression respond to tricyclic antidepressants in lower-than-usual therapeutic dosages. Antidepressants that are less anticholinergic, such as desipramine or nortriptyline, should be used to avoid central anticholinergic toxicity. Once treatable organic causes have been ruled out, florid organic manic episodes can be successfully treated with antipsychotics and lithium carbonate. Since

some AIDS patients appear to be more vulnerable to the central nervous system toxicity of lithium, it is prudent to aim for an initial serum blood level of 0.5 to 1.0 mEq/l. Carbamazepine is effective in treating mania but its ability to produce leukopenia can make it a problematic drug to use in patients with low white blood counts. Apart from psychotic features associated with AIDS dementia complex, acute psychoses also can occur. An individual with new onset of psychosis requires immediate psychiatric evaluation and treatment.

Psychiatric diagnosis is difficult in AIDS patients because of the combination of organic mental disorders and strong emotional reactions to lethal illness. These aspects are not mutually exclusive and when they

Table V Mini-Mental State Exam*

Patient_______________________________________

Examiner _____________________________________

Date____

	Maximum Score	Score
Orientation	10	
What is the (year), (season), (day of month), (month), (day of week)? (1 point for each)		____
Where are we: (state), (county), (town), (hospital), (floor)? (1 point for each)		____
Registration	3	
Name 3 objects: 1 second to say each. Then ask the patient all 3 after you have said them. Give 1 point for each correct answer. Then repeat them until he learns all 3. Count trials and record.		____
Trials		
Attention And Calculation	5	
Serials 7s. 1 point for each correct. Stop after 5 answers. Alternatively spell "world" backwards.		____
Recall	3	
Ask for the 3 objects repeated above. Give 1 point for each correct.		____
Language	9	
Name a pencil and a watch (2 points).		____
Repeat the following: "No ifs, ands, or buts" (1 point)		
Follow a three-stage command: "Take a paper in your right hand, fold it in half, and put it on the floor." (3 points)		____
Read and obey the following: "Close your eyes." (1 point)		____
Write a sentence (1 point)		____
Copy this design (1 point)		____
Total Score	30	

Scoring†:   24-30 Normal
                  20-23 Mild dementia
                  10-19 Moderate dementia
                  < 10 Severe dementia

*See Folstein reference in "Additional Reading" section

†Education and sensory/motor deficits are defined in the first full paragraph, this page.

coexist, both need to be addressed in the overall treatment plan. An organic cause of mental status changes should be suspected in all HIV-infected patients before concluding that the symptoms are solely part of a functional syndrome, such as adjustment disorder.

The opinions, conclusions and proposals in this paper are those of the authors and may not represent the views of the Robert Wood Johnson Foundation or the Veterans Administration.

Additional Reading

Anders, K. H., Guerra, W. F., Tomiyasu, U., Verity, M. A., Vinters, H. V. 1986. The neuropathology of AIDS. UCLA experience and review. *Am J Pathol* 124:537-558.

Armstrong, D., Gold, J.W.M., Dryjanski, J. *et al*. 1985. Treatment of infections in patients with the acquired immunodeficiency syndrome. *Ann Int Med* 103:738.

Centers for Disease Control. 1987. Classification system for human immunodeficiency virus (HIV) infection in children under 13 years of age. *Morbid Mortal Weekly Rep* 36:225-36.

Centers for Disease Control. 1986. Classification system for human T-lymphotropic virus type III/lymphadenopathy virus type III infections. *Morbid Mortal Weekly Rep* 35:334-9.

Folstein, M.F., Folstein, S.E., McHugh, P.R. 1975. "Mini-mental state"—A practical method for grading the cognitive state of patients for the clinician. *J Psychiatric Res* 12:189-198.

Levy, R.M., Bredesen, D.E., Rosenblum, M.L. 1985. Neurological manifestations of the acquired immunodeficiency syndrome (AIDS): Experience at UCSF and review of the literature. *J Neurosurg* 62:475-495.

Navia, B.A., Jordan, B.D., Price, R.W. 1986. The AIDS dementia complex: I. Clinical features. *Ann Neurol* 19:517-524.

Wolcott, D.L., Fawzy, F.I., Pasnau, R.O. 1985. Acquired immune deficiency syndrome (AIDS) and consultation-liaison psychiatry. *Gen Hosp Psychiatry* 7:280-292.

CME Examination

Complete this test and return the enclosed answer sheet in the envelope provided with $15 to be eligible for 4 hours of Category I CME credit. Transcripts will be mailed to participants with a passing grade of 70 percent or more answers correct.

INSTRUCTIONS: Choose the one best answer.

Epidemiology

1. Which of the following factors is generally accepted as carrying a risk of transmitting human immunodeficiency virus (HIV) from an infected to an uninfected person?

   A. Mosquitoes

   B. Breast feeding

   C. Sharing drinking glasses

   D. All of the above

   E. None of the above

2. Considering the occurrence of reported cases of AIDS in the United States and the Pacific Northwest, which of the following statements is false?

   A. Nationally, AIDS cases in IV drug abusers outnumber cases in homosexual and bisexua. men.

   B. Cases attributed to heterosexual transmission are relatively more common nationally than in the Pacific Northwest.

   C. To date, most heterosexually acquired AIDS cases in women have occurred in the sexual partners of IV drug abusers.

   D. Most children with AIDS acquired HIV infection *in utero* or perinatally from an infected mother.

   E. None of the above

3. Which of the following sequences best characterizes the prevalence of HIV infection (not overt AIDS) in various risk groups in the Pacific Northwest?

   A. Hemophiliacs > IV drug abusers > Homosexual men

   B. IV drug abusers > Heterosexual patients in sexually transmitted disease (STD) clinics > Hemophiliacs

   C. Homosexual and bisexual men > Heterosexual patients in STD clinics > IV drug abusers

   D. Homosexual and bisexual men > IV drug abusers > Heterosexual patients of STD clinics

   E. None of the above

4. Which of the following statements accurately characterizes the AIDS epidemic in the United States?

   A. More AIDS cases occur in 20- to 29-year-olds than in any other age group.

   B. About 20 percent of reported AIDS cases have been in women.

   C. Whites with AIDS outnumber members of all other ethnic groups with AIDS.

   D. A cumulative total of approximately 100,000 AIDS cases is expected through 1991.

   E. None of the above

Public Health

5. Physicians should encourage "safe sex" practices for:

   A. Homosexual and bisexual men

   B. Prostitutes and IV drug abusers

   C. Sexually active persons outside monogamous relationships

   D. Those who test seropositive for HIV infection

   E. All of the above

6. One-to-one counseling:

   A. Is especially important for high-risk populations

   B. Has less impact than information addressed to general audiences

   C. Is secondary to testing in achieving control of HIV infection

   D. Is not part of a primary-care physician's role

   E. Is rarely sought by persons at low risk

7. Partner notification:

   A. Is certainly cost-effective within high-risk groups

   B. May be useful for exposed partners who are unaware of their risk

   C. Is futile in AIDS because no current treatment eradicates HIV

   D. Is used to control other communicable diseases

   E. B and D

HIV and Related Retroviruses

8. Human immunodeficiency viruses (HIV-1 and -2) belong to the lentivirus subfamily of retroviruses and are distinct from both HTLV-I and HTLV-II, which belong to the oncovirus subfamily of retroviruses.

   A. True

   B. False

9. HIV-2 may be more closely related to HIV-1 than it is to the simian immunodeficiency virus (SIV).

   A. True

   B. False

10. Which of the following statements about HIV is false?

    A. HIV is a retrovirus characterized by the presence of reverse transcriptase.

    B. The envelope of HIV is studded with a virus-encoded glycoprotein that contains the attachment site for the CD4 T-cell receptor.

    C. The HIV provirus may either integrate into the host cell genome or remain in an extrachromosomal form.

    D. Because HIV is an enveloped virus it can withstand the harsh environmental conditions imposed by detergents, heat and drying.

11. Which of the following statements about the physiopathology of HIV is false?

    A. Unlike HTLV-I, HIV does not transform infected cells.

    B. HIV depletes the CD4 T-cell population through the fusion of infected with uninfected CD4 T-cells.

    C. The envelope gene of HIV demonstrates areas of hypervariability.

    D. The monocyte-macrophage is not infected by HIV because it both lacks the CD4 receptor and is capable of inactivating ingested HIV particles.

Laboratory Diagnosis

12. Confirmatory tests for screening ELISA tests include:

    A. Western blot

    B. Radioimmunoprecipitation

    C. Immunofluorescence

    D. Use of recombinant proteins in ELISA tests

    E. All of the above

13. Detection of HIV antigen has been used to:

    A. Monitor viral cultures *in vitro*

    B. Detect virus in serum very early and very late in the course of HIV infection

    C. Follow disease course

    D. A & C

    E. A, B & C

14. Which of the following statements about HIV infection is false?

    A. Antigenemia precedes the development of an antibody response to the glycoprotein (gp41) and core (p24) proteins of HIV.

    B. Following exposure to HIV, most persons will develop an antibody response to the various HIV proteins by three months.

    C. In some HIV-infected patients, a drop in p24 antibody is associated with a concomitant rise in p24 antigen.

    D. HIV-seropositive patients should be advised that the presence of HIV antibody does not necessarily mean that they will be infectious.

15. Which of the following statements about HIV culture is false?

    A. HIV can be isolated from infected lymphocytes by cocultivation with lymphocytes from a normal person.

    B. HIV culture of peripheral blood lymphocytes, body fluids, and tissues may be required to establish HIV infection in infants less than 15 months of age.

    C. The rate of HIV isolation and p24 antigen detection from plasma of patients with AIDS and AIDS-related complex is higher than from plasma of asymptomatic seropositive persons. This suggests that body fluids (for example, blood) from patients with AIDS and ARC may be more infectious than similar fluids from asymptomatic seropositive persons.

    D. Because HIV culture is generally quite sensitive, very specific, and inexpensive, it is suitable for the routine diagnosis of HIV infection.

Clinical Manifestations

16. The most common cause of dementia in persons with HIV infection is thought to be:

    A. Central nervous system lymphoma

    B. Toxoplasmosis

    C. HIV infection

    D. Cryptococcal meningitis

    E. Cytomegalovirus encephalitis

17. The spectrum of illness caused by HIV includes all of the following except:

    A. Asymptomatic state

    B. Immunodeficiency

    C. Dementia

    D. Peptic ulcer disease

    E. Aseptic meningitis

18. Lesions of Kaposi's sarcoma are typically not:

    A. Violaceous

    B. Painful

    C. Multicolored

    D. Nodular

    E. Macular

19. The most common serious infection associated with AIDS in the United States is:

    A. Oral candidiasis

    B. Cryptococcal meningitis

    C. Central nervous system toxoplasmosis

    D. Pulmonary tuberculosis

    E. *Pneumocystis carinii* pneumonia

20. Recognized symptoms of primary HIV infection include all of the following except:

    A. Dyspnea

    B. Skin rash

    C. Lymphadenopathy

    D. Fever

    E. Headache

Anti-Retroviral Chemotherapy

21. Which of the following potential targets for inhibiting HIV replication has been the mechanism of action of several anti-retroviral compounds including zidovudine?

    A. Inhibition of attachment and blockage of HIV into the T4 cell

    B. Prevention of intracellular uncoating

    C. Inhibition of reverse transcriptase

    D. Inhibition of HIV replication (integration of post-transcription processing)

    E. Inhibition of release (budding) of HIV from T4 cell

22. All the following drug combinations are synergistic *in vitro* except:

    A. Zidovudine and alpha interferon

    B. Zidovudine and acyclovir

    C. Ribavirin and Foscarnet™ (PFA)

    D. Ribavirin and zidovudine

    E. Lymphoblastoid interferon and zidovudine

23. Which of the following anti-HIV agents is paired with an adverse reaction not associated with that agent?

    A. Suramin and adrenal insufficiency

    B. HPA-23 and thrombocytopenia

    C. Zidovudine and bone marrow suppression

    D. Foscarnet™ (PFA) and hepatitis

    E. Ribavirin and reversible anemia

24. Which of the following statements regarding zidovudine is incorrect?

    A. The FDA-approved maximum dosage is 200 mg orally q 4 hours.

    B. Anemia secondary to zidovudine usually appears in the first 72 hours.

    C. Zidovudine appears to penetrate the blood-brain barrier with cerebrospinal fluid ranging from 10 percent to 50 percent of plasma concentrations.

    D. Acetaminophen, rifampin and cimetidine may inhibit zidovudine's metabolism and therefore should not be co-administered.

    E. Patients with asymptomatic HIV infection or persistent generalized lymphadenopathy are currently not eligible to receive FDA-approved zidovudine.

Psychosocial Aspects

25. Which of the following groups of sexual practices is the least safe with regard to HIV transmission?

    A. Receptive anal intercourse without a condom

    B. Genital manipulation; french (wet) kissing

    C. Fellatio but stopping before climax; anal intercourse with a condom

    D. Vaginal intercourse

26. Which of the following questions is most likely to elicit the most clinically relevant information for assessing risk of HIV infection from sexual practices?

    A. "Do you consider yourself heterosexual or homosexual?"

    B. "Have you ever done anything that might have placed you at risk for AIDS?"

    C. "In the last 10 years, have you engaged in unprotected anal intercourse with someone you were not absolutely sure was not infected?"

27. Which of the following will help ameliorate some of the fears of death and dying in persons with AIDS?

    A. Allowing the person with AIDS to exercise as much control as possible over treatment decisions

    B. Physical contact, such as therapeutic touch

    C. Referral to support groups and other AIDS-related social service agencies

    D. Helping the patient get his/her affairs in order soon after the diagnosis

    E. All of the above

28. Waves of extreme anxiety that alternate with denial and emotional "numbing" are most frequently experienced during which phase of psychological adaptation to AIDS or disabling AIDS-related complex (ARC)?

    A. Initial

    B. Middle or transitional

    C. Terminal

    D. None of the above

Infection Control

29. The San Francisco AIDS Task Force evaluated several approaches for screening and taking infection precautions with patients being admitted to hospitals. Which answer reflects its recommendation?

    A. Screen all admissions for HIV and take precautions only with those who have positive test results.

    B. Screen only surgical patients and take precautions only with those who have positive test results.

    C. Screen all gay men, IV drug abusers, hemophiliacs and sexual contacts of members of these groups and take precautions only with them.

    D. Screen only for clinical indications but take precautions with all patients.

30. Of the nine health care workers believed to have acquired HIV on the job, what proportion had a preceding puncture with a contaminated needle?

    A. 1/9

    B. 4/9

    C. 6/9

    D. 9/9

31. Dentists and other personnel should use protective barriers when performing invasive procedures for which patients?

    A. Gay men, hemophiliacs and IV drug abusers

    B. Any patients believed to be at high risk for AIDS

    C. Diagnosed cases of AIDS and AIDS-related complex (ARC)

    D. All patients

32. Three infections commonly seen in AIDS patients that could potentially cause nosocomial infections in health care workers are:

    A. Tuberculosis, herpes simplex and varicella zoster

    B. *Pneumocystis*, cryptococcosis and toxoplasmosis

    C. Toxoplasmosis, candidiasis and *Mycobacterium avium-intracellulare*

Global Perspective

33. Infection with certain sexually transmitted pathogens has been implicated in sexual transmission of HIV. Prominent among these is/are:

    A. *Phthirus pubis* (crab lice) infestation

    B. Human papilloma virus (genital warts)

    C. *Haemophilus ducreyi* (chancroid)

    D. *Molluscum contagiosum*

    E. All of the above

34. Given the epidemiology of AIDS in Africa, which of the following control measures would you institute?

    A. Blood bank screening

    B. Education of health care personnel regarding appropriate sterilization techniques for reusable needles and syringes

    C. Serologic testing of high-risk populations

    D. Health education and condom distribution for high-risk individuals (for example, prostitutes and other persons with multiple sexual partners)

    E. All of the above

35. Which of the following statements is true?

    A. The country with the largest number of AIDS cases reported to the World Health Organization is Zaire.

    B. AIDS has been reported from every continent except Asia.

    C. Given that AIDS is a pandemic disease, a policy of screening immigrants for HIV antibody would have a major impact on limiting the burden of HIV infection in the United States.

    D. The World Health Organization predicts that as many as 100 million persons worldwide will be infected by 1991.

    E. A study in Kinshasa showed an association between malaria and HIV infection, suggesting that insect vectors may be important in the spread of the AIDS epidemic in tropical settings.

36. What factor(s) may account for the predominance of heterosexual transmission as the primary mode of spread of HIV in Africa?

    A. Sexually transmitted diseases, epidemic in many parts of Africa

    B. Patterns of prostitution

    C. Disruption of family units and traditional cultures through rural-urban migration of the male work force

    D. None of the above

    E. All of the above

Prospects in Anti-Retroviral Chemotherapy for Treatment of HIV Infection

by Teresa A. Tartaglione, Pharm.D., and Lawrence Corey, M.D.

The complex biology of the human immunodeficiency virus (HIV), the fact that it infects a wide variety of cells and anatomic sites, and its ability to both latently and productively infect lymphocytes and neuronal cells present enormous challenges for any chemotherapeutic agent. Multiple strategies to inhibit HIV may be needed. Our review focuses on current strategies to treat HIV infection and provides guidelines for the primary physician for use of anti-retroviral agents.

Targets for antiviral activity against HIV

The replicative ("life") cycle of HIV follows a set pattern of virus attachment, entry into the host cell, virus uncoating, viral replication, and virus assembly and release from the cell. Each step represents a potential target for antiviral attack (Table I, Figure 1).

Dr. Tartaglione is an assistant professor of pharmacy at the University of Washington. Dr. Corey is a UW professor of laboratory medicine, microbiology and medicine.

Inhibition of attachment or entry of HIV into a cell has theoretical appeal because such a strategy would prevent development both of latent and of productive infection. Attachment can be inhibited by human monoclonal antibodies directed against the cell receptors (T4 molecules) to which the virus attaches. Compounds that block the cell receptor, or alter the virus envelope glycoprotein by which the virus attaches to the cell receptor, are undergoing clinical investigation. Peptide T, a 10-amino-acid peptide, binds to a region on the T4 molecule and appears to prevent HIV from entering cells. AL 7,2,1 is a combination of fatty acids which are taken up by infected cells and alter the composition of the virus envelope glycoprotein, resulting in inhibition of HIV replication *in vitro*. AL 7,2,1 is just entering phase I clinical trials.

After attachment and entry, the next step that could be inhibited in theory is the intracellular uncoating of the virus. No compounds that inhibit this viral process have yet entered clinical trials. However, several compounds have been developed that inhibit the next steps, which involve viral RNA and DNA replication. Reverse transcriptase is a viral enzyme that is essential to HIV replication but has no essential mammalian cell function. Inhibition of reverse transcriptase, therefore, should act selectively on retroviruses. Zidovudine (formerly known as azidothymidine or AZT) appears to be the prototype of compounds with this mechanism of action.

Other potential targets for inhibiting HIV replication include viral integration into the host cell DNA; post-transcription processing of viral messenger RNA; and assembly and release of the virus. Several HIV gene products enhance viral replication but not cellular DNA replication. Inhibitors of these gene products may decrease the number of infectious virions circulating in the body. Inhibitors of the latter steps of viral replication have not yet been developed. Finally, the anti-retroviral effect of interferon appears to be on the release of HIV from infected cells. Clinical trials of interferon as a single agent for HIV treatment have been disappointing thus far.

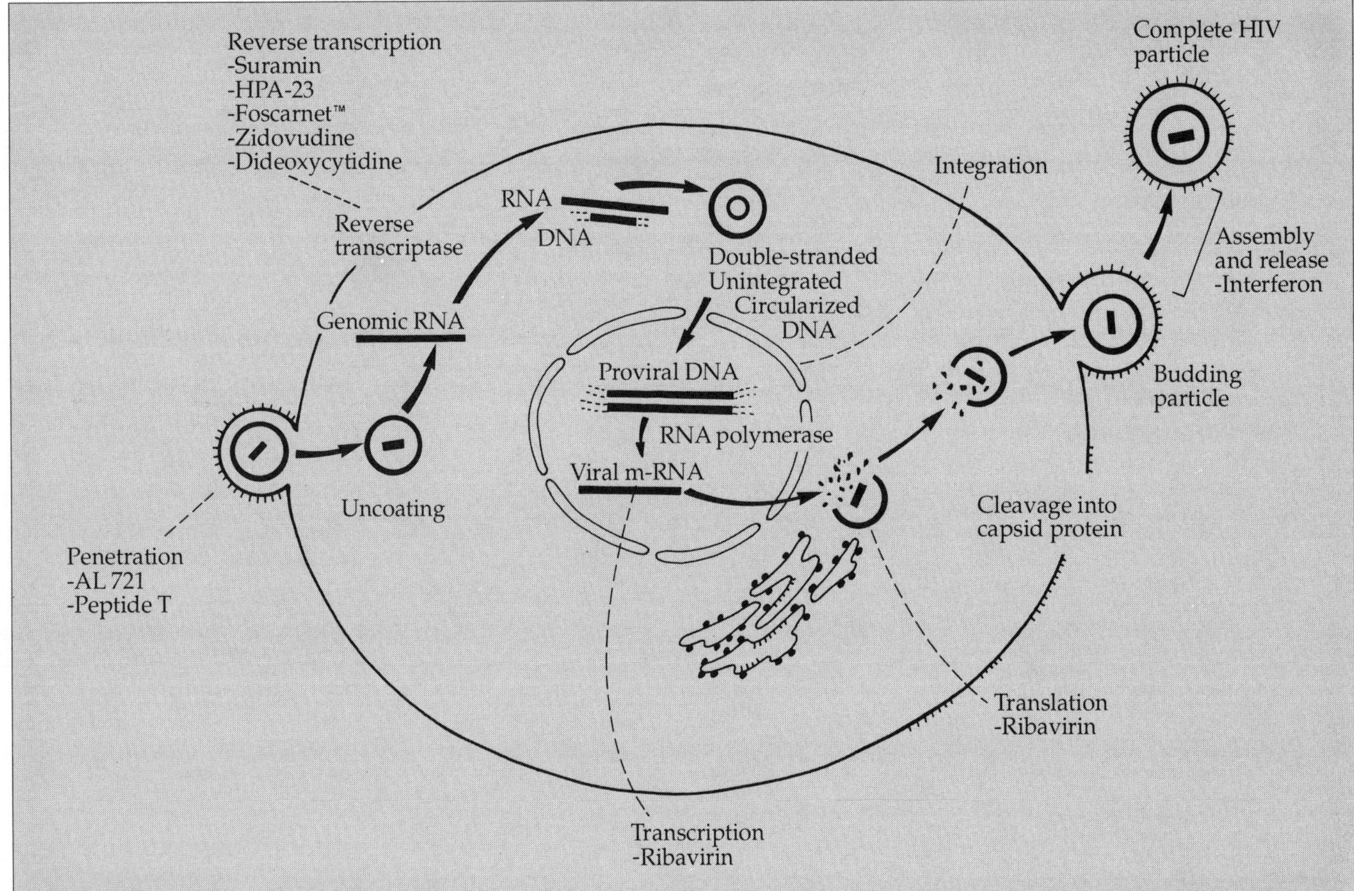

FIGURE 1. The replication cycle of human immunodeficiency virus and possible sites of drug action. Reproduced with permission from Hirsch. Prospects of Therapy for Infections with Human T-Lymphotropic Virus Type III. *Ann Intern Med* 1987; 103:752.

Antiviral combinations may be more effective than a single antiviral agent alone, especially if the drugs have different mechanisms of action and appear additive or synergistic *in vitro* and/or in animal models. Combinations of antivirals such as zidovudine and interferon are under active clinical investigation.

Agents that have been shown to potentiate the host's immune system *in vitro*—such as interleukin-2, inosine pranobex, gamma interferon and levamisole—have been suggested as potential therapies for persons with acquired immunodeficiency syndrome (AIDS) and AIDS-related complex (ARC). Combination chemotherapy with antiviral agents and these immune modulators also has been proposed.

Concepts for design and conduct of clinical trials for HIV infection

Because no practical animal models for treatment of HIV infection are available, several criteria have been proposed to evaluate the effects of potential chemotherapeutic agents for HIV. These include: a reduction in the ability to isolate virus during and after therapy; restoration of some of the immunologic dysfunctions seen in AIDS, such as an increase in the number of circulating CD4+ cells; restoration of cutaneous hypersensitivity; a decrease in the clinical manifestations of disease, including fever, diarrhea and weight loss; and prevention of opportunistic infections.

The most extensively tested of the antiviral compounds that inhibit HIV *in vitro* are summarized in Table II. In nearly all *in-vitro* systems tested, HIV replication resumes when the antiviral drug is removed from HIV-infected cells, indicating that the drugs inhibit productive viral replication but don't cure the cell of latently infected provirus. This implies that chronic administration of these drugs will be required. Because HIV is usually present in the central nervous system in most infected persons, antiviral drugs for HIV infection must be able to cross the blood-brain barrier.

Selected antiviral agents with activity against HIV

Suramin

Suramin, an anti-parasitic agent used clinically to treat East African trypanosomiasis and onchocerciasis, was the first drug reported to have *in-vitro* activity against HIV. HIV was inhibited *in vitro* by a concentration of 100 mcg/ml, achievable with a one-gram intravenous dose. Clinical trials of suramin for HIV treatment were undertaken in early 1984.

Although isolation of HIV from peripheral blood lymphocytes was transiently decreased, side effects were frequent and severe, and there was no clinical or immunologic improvement nor reduction in the frequency of opportunistic infections. This first report of HIV antiviral therapy illustrated the necessity of controlled clinical trials of AIDS antivirals and showed that even well-researched agents may cause adverse clinical effects previously unrecognized in HIV-infected persons.

HPA-23

Ammonium 21-tungsto-9-antimoniate (HPA-23) inhibits reverse transcriptase *in vitro* at concentrations of approximately 30 mcg/ml. This drug garnered much attention when it was used by actor Rock Hudson. However, despite phase I trials initiated two years ago, little is known about its potential antiviral effects or its pharmacology. The drug is poorly absorbed orally, and its penetration into the cerebrospinal fluid is unknown.

In France, 47 patients have received intravenous doses of HPA-23 ranging from 50 to 200 mg/day, with some evidence of *in-vivo* inhibition of HIV replication. However, 33 of the 47 developed thrombocytopenia and many had hepatic transaminase elevations. Little observable clinical improvement was noted. These limited data suggest HPA-23 is fairly toxic and lacks dramatic antiviral effects.

Ribavirin

Ribavirin is a synthetic purine nucleoside that is active *in vitro* against a broad spectrum of DNA and RNA viruses, including HIV. It has been widely tested for treatment of influenza A and B, and is licensed in the United States in aerosol form for treatment of respiratory syncytial virus infections. Orally, it decreases mortality from lassa fever virus infection. Ribavirin's mechanism of action is not completely understood, though it is a competitive inhibitor of reverse transcriptase and interferes with viral mRNA synthesis.

HIV replication is partially suppressed at concentrations of 50 to 100 mcg/ml. Single doses of 600 mg to 2400 mg produce peak serum concentrations ranging from 1.2 to 3.0 mcg/ml after oral administration and from 10 to 40 mcg/ml after intravenous administration. It has excellent cerebrospinal fluid penetration.

Trials of systemic ribavirin in HIV infection were initiated in early 1985. Men with HIV infections tolerated ribavirin well; a reversible reduction in hemoglobin was its major toxic effect. In a controlled trial involving 163 patients with generalized lymphadenopathy, 107 patients received either 600 or 800 mg of ribavirin orally once per day, and 56 received placebo. Initial reports indicated that 18 percent of placebo recipients progressed to AIDS, versus 11 percent of the recipients of 600 mg of ribavirin and none of the recipients of 800 mg. However, it appears that the placebo and 600-mg groups had a lower number of circulating T4 cells prior to entry, a parameter that we now know markedly affects the rate of progression to AIDS. When data are stratified by T4 count, there is no evidence that ribavirin decreases progression of patients with HIV-associated lymphadenopathy. An identical trial in ARC patients has not shown any benefits thus far.

Phosphonoformate

Trisodium phosphonoformate hexahydrate (PFA, Foscarnet™) was first synthesized in 1924 and is structurally related to pyrophosphate. PFA inhibits a wide range of DNA and RNA polymerases, including those of all herpes viruses (herpes simplex virus, cytomegalovirus, Epstein-Barr virus and varicella zoster virus), hepatitis B virus and HIV. Specifically, PFA appears to interact with nucleic acid polymerases at the site where pyrophosphate is released during elongation of the DNA or RNA chain. PFA inhibits HIV reverse transcriptase at concentrations (approximately 1 uM of PFA) that do not affect cell DNA synthesis.

Table I Possible Targets for Therapeutic Intervention in Stages of HIV Replication

Stage	Possible Intervention
Binding to target cell	Antibodies to virus or cellular receptor
Entry into target cell and uncoating RNA	Drugs that block fusion or interfere with retroviral uncoating
Transcription of RNA to DNA by reverse transcriptase	Reverse transcriptase inhibitors
Degradation of RNA by RNase activity (encoded by viral *pol* gene)	RNase H inhibitors
Integration of DNA into host genome	Agents that inhibit polymerase-mediated integration may be found.
Transcription of DNA to RNA	Specific inhibitors of retrovirus transcription have not been developed.
Translation of RNA	Inhibitors of genes that enhance retrovirus translation, such as *tat*III or *art*/*trs*
Viral component production and assembly	Inhibitors or modifiers of glycosylation of viral proteins
Viral budding	Interferons; antibodies to a viral antigen

Reprinted by permission from *Nature*, Vol. 325, pp. 773-778. Copyright (c) 1987 Macmillan Journals Limited.

PFA currently is available only as an intravenous product. It has been tested in humans most extensively as a topical drug for herpes simplex virus infections and as intravenous therapy in immunosuppressed patients with severe cytomegalovirus infection. In the latter studies, a dosage of 20 mg/kg/24 hours was administered as a continuous infusion. Plasma concentrations ranged from 250 to 500 uM (75 to 150 mcg/ml) during the infusion period. Most of the drug is eliminated unchanged in the urine with an estimated serum elimination half-life of six hours. PFA appears to penetrate into the cerebrospinal fluid in patients with and without meningeal inflammation.

Pilot studies with PFA in patients with AIDS and ARC are under way in both the United States and Europe. Preliminary results indicate some clinical improvement, return of delayed type hypersensitivity, and negative cultures for the virus during therapy in several patients. Clinical trials with PFA administered daily as an intravenous infusion will start in the United States in late 1987.

Zidovudine (azidothymidine or AZT)

Activity and Pharmacology

Zidovudine is a clinically effective reverse transcriptase inhibitor of HIV and is marketed under the name Retrovir™. Zidovudine is a thymidine analog in which the 3' hydroxy (-OH) group is replaced by an azido (NH3) group. At concentrations of 0.13 mcg/ml or less, zidovudine inhibits 90 percent of detectable HIV replication *in vitro*. *In vivo*, zidovudine is converted by cellular enzymes to a triphosphate form (zidovudine-TP) that is subsequently utilized by HIV reverse transcriptase (Figure 2). When zidovudine-TP is incorporated into the growing DNA chain of HIV, the DNA synthesis is terminated.

A series of pharmacokinetic studies of oral zidovudine showed that serum concentrations averaged 0.62 mcg/ml (range 0.05 to 1.46 mcg/ml) following chronic oral administration of 250 mg every four hours (3 to 5.4 mg/kg). Following oral administration, zidovudine bioavailability is approximately 70 percent due to drug metabolism in its first pass through the liver. Plasma protein binding is 34 to 38 percent. Zidovudine's mean terminal half-life is approximately 1.1 hours. Renal clearance of zidovudine is estimated to be 400 ml/min/70 kg, approximately 20 percent of total body clearance. The 5'-glucuronide conjugate of zidovudine (glucuronylzidovudine) is a major inactive plasma and urinary metabolite. Glucuronylzidovudine is rapidly cleared from plasma with a half-life of approximately one hour. The cerebrospinal fluid/plasma concentration ratio was 0.15 in one patient 1.8 hours following a 2-mg/kg oral dose. Two to four hours after a 5-mg/kg intravenous dose, the ratio was 0.64. Our experience with 19 patients revealed that most cerebrospinal fluid concentrations (range 0.028-0.183 mcg/ml) were below inhibitory concentrations.

Clinical efficacy and toxicity

A phase III, randomized, double-blind, placebo-controlled trial of zidovudine's ability to decrease AIDS morbidity and mortality was conducted at 12 U.S. medical centers. One-hundred-sixty AIDS patients and 121 patients with advanced ARC were studied for an average of four and one-half months. All AIDS patients had recovered from their first episode of *Pneumocystis carinii* pneumonia diagnosed within the previous four months. Patients were given placebo or 250 mg of zidovudine every four hours around the clock. Dosages were reduced to 100 mg every four hours or permanently discontinued if toxicity developed. After four months of therapy, 19 deaths had occurred in the placebo group and one in the zidovudine group (p<.001). All deaths were due to opportunistic infections or other complications of HIV infection. Because of this decrease in mortality in the zidovudine group, the trial was discontinued for ethical reasons.

In addition to a lower mortality, patients who received zidovudine experienced better performance, better neuropsychiatric function, maintained their body weight, and had fewer and less severe symptoms associated with HIV infection. Preliminary data also suggested some reduction in circulating amounts of HIV core protein (p24) with zidovudine-treated patients.

Zidovudine did, however, produce some serious side effects. Granulocytopenia and anemia necessitated dose reduction or drug discontinuation in 49 of the 143 (34 percent) patients (Table III). Blood transfusions were required for 31 percent of the patients receiving zidovudine and for 11 percent of those on placebo. In general, decreases in hemoglobin and neutrophils occurred during the second month of therapy and appeared to be reversible if the dose was decreased or the drug discontinued. Other side effects reported with zidovudine include rashes, pruritus, nausea, headache, mild confusion and other neurotoxicity (Table IV). Complaints of headache or confusion may precede severe neurotoxicity and should be monitored closely.

Practical guidelines for administration

On the basis of this information, the Food and Drug Administration (FDA) approved zidovudine in March 1987 for management of adult patients with AIDS and advanced ARC who have a history of cytologically confirmed *Pneumocystis carinii* pneumonia or an absolute T4 lymphocyte count of less than 200/mm3 in their peripheral blood. Bimonthly screening of T4 counts will allow patients with borderline counts (>200 but <500) to become eligible for zidovudine as soon as possible. The recommended starting dose is 200 mg orally every four hours around the clock, with dosage adjustment - frequently required during the course of therapy as dictated by toxicity. At present it

Table II Antivirals Active Against HIV *In Vitro*

Agent	Anti-HIV Concentration	Achievable Serum Level	Proposed Mechanism of Action
Suramin	suppression at 50 mcg/ml; inhibition at 100-1,000 mcg/ml	> 100 mcg/ml	reverse transcriptase inhibition
Ribavirin	suppression at 10-100 mcg/ml	1-3 mcg/ml	reverse transcriptase inhibition
HPA-23	ID50* 30 mcg/ml	N/A†	reverse transcriptase inhibition
Alpha Interferon	suppression at 4-64 U/ml; inhibition at 256-1,064 U/ml	50-300 U/ml	inhibits budding
PFA	suppression at 132 uM; inhibition at 680 uM	100-450 uM	reverse transcriptase inhibition
Zidovudine (AZT)	0.13-2.7 mcg/ml	0.5-3.0 mcg/ml	reverse transcriptase inhibition; DNA chain termination
AL 7,2,1	ED50‡ 100 mcg/ml ED90 1,000 mcg/ml	N/A	alteration of viral envelope
Dideoxycytidine	0.1-0.5 mcg/ml	0.02-0.4 mcg/ml	reverse transcriptase inhibition; DNA chain termination

*ID50 = the median infective dose; the amount of pathogenic microorganisms that will produce infection in 50 percent of test subjects.

†N/A = not available

‡ED50/90 = the median effective dose; a dose that produces effects in 50/90 percent of a population.

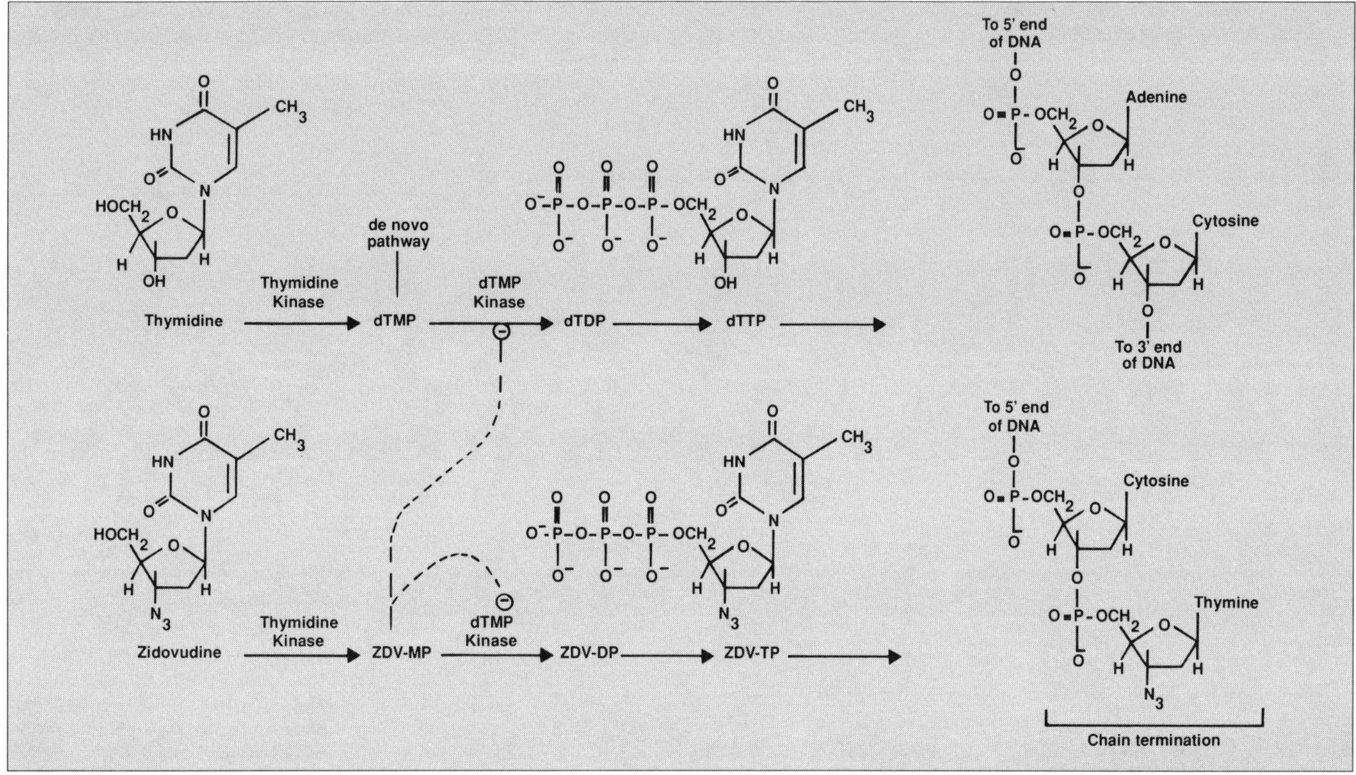

FIGURE 2. The intracellular metabolism of thymidine (top) and zidovudine (ZDV) at bottom.

(A) ZDV-MP interferes with the phosphorylation of dTMP by competitive substrate inhibition. Cells exposed to ZDV may have high levels of dTMP and decreased levels of dTTP, which may be one factor that contributes to the drug's toxicity.

(B) The thymidine pathway at top results in a normal DNA chain. When ZDV-TP (bottom) is bound by a DNA polymerase and incorporated onto the growing 3' end of a DNA chain, the subsequent 5'→3' phosphodiester linkages necessary to add other nucleosides cannot form, and the chain is terminated.

Reprinted by permission of *The New England Journal of Medicine*, Vol. 316, p. 561-2, 1987.

is best to consult with persons experienced in zidovudine use. Hematologic parameters should be carefully monitored at least every two weeks; reductions in hemoglobin may occur as early as two to four weeks, whereas granulocytopenia often is not observed until weeks six to eight.

Patients whose hemoglobin concentration drops to less than 7.5 gm/dl should have zidovudine discontinued until the hemoglobin value is at least 9.5 gm/dl. We recommend that patients not be transfused at this time unless their cardiovascular status is compromised or their hemoglobin concentration fails to improve by at least 1 gm/dl within seven days of zidovudine discontinuation. If transfusion is performed, zidovudine may be restarted in seven days if the hemoglobin concentration has stabilized. In either case, zidovudine should be reinstated at half the initial dose (for example, 100 mg q 4 hours). If a patient continues to exhibit low or falling hemoglobin concentrations, we currently continue the medication if transfusion requirements are less than four units every 21 days or if the hemoglobin concentration does not fall below 6.5 gm/dl on two consecutive episodes at least one week apart despite blood transfusions. If persistent, life-threatening anemia develops (hemoglobin .5 gm/dl), we discontinue zidovudine permanently. This occurs in 10 to 20 percent of patients.

For other severe, zidovudine-induced toxicities, including granulocytopenia (polymorphonuclear leukocytes 500-750/m3), we discontinue zidovudine until baseline values return. Zidovudine is then restarted at 100 mg q 4 hours. If severe toxicity resumes, we recommend discontinuing zidovudine permanently. We currently recommend that you confer with a person experienced with zidovudine use when toxicity occurs.

Limited information is available regarding the interaction of other drugs with zidovudine. Co-administration of zidovudine with agents that produce hematologic, nephrotoxic or cytotoxic effects (dapsone, pentamidine, amphotericin B, flucytosine, vincristine, vinblastine, adriamycin, interferon) may potentiate the risk of toxicity. Drugs that may competitively inhibit glucuronidation should be avoided. These include acetaminophen, rifampin, cimetidine, ranitidine, flurazepam, indomethacin and probenecid. Acetaminophen used concomitantly with zidovudine appears to enhance the risk of granulocytopenia. The current recommendation is to temporarily discontinue zidovudine if an opportunistic infection develops. Little information regarding additive toxicity is available for trimethoprim-

Table III Hematologic Side Effects in Patients with AIDS and AIDS-Related Complex Receiving Zidovudine (AZT) or Placebo

| | Pretreatment T4 Levels | | | |
| | < 200/mm3 | | >200/mm3 | |
Abnormality	Zidovudine (n=113)	Placebo (n=105)	Zidovudine (n=30)	Placebo (n=30)
Granulocytopenia:				
< 750/mm3	47%	10%	10%	3%
50% reduction in baseline value	55%	19%	40%	13%
Anemia:				
Hgb < 7.5 g/dl	30%	6%	3%	0%
25% reduction in baseline value	45%	14%	10%	10%

From Burroughs Wellcome Co. Retrovir™ package insert; March 1987.

Table IV Side Effects Profile of AIDS and ARC Patients Receiving Either Zidovudine (AZT) or Placebo

Adverse Event	Zidovudine* (n=144) %	Placebo (n=137) %
Headache	42	37
Fever	16	12
Malaise	8	7
Diaphoresis	5	4
Myalgia	8	2
Nausea	46	18
Vomiting	6	3
Diarrhea	12	18
Anorexia	11	8
GI Pain	20	19
Dizziness	6	4
Insomnia	5	1
Paresthesia	6	3
Somnolence	8	9

*Initial starting dose of zidovudine was 250 mg orally q 4 hrs.
From Burroughs Wellcome Co. Retrovir™ package insert; March 1987.

sulfamethoxazole, pyrimethamine and others. Chronic administration of other medications with zidovudine has not been systematically studied and should be avoided when possible.

Patients taking these medications should be followed by specialists experienced with the clinical presentations of AIDS and the complications of zidovudine therapy.

Dideoxycytidine

2′, 3′—dideoxycytidine is another nucleoside analog that is similar in structure to zidovudine. It appears to be a more potent inhibitor than zidovudine of the replication and cytopathic effect of HIV in some in-vitro systems. Concentrations ranging from 0.5 uM (0.1 mcg/ml) to 2 uM (0.425 mcg/ml) inhibit HIV growth and prevent expression of the p24 core protein in T-cell lines. Preliminary data from a phase I trial demonstrated plasma concentrations of 0.02 to 0.06 mcg/ml and 0.2 to 0.4 mcg/ml following single, one-hour intravenous infusions of 0.03 mg/kg and 0.25 mg/kg, respectively. The elimination half-life of dideoxycytidine is approximately one hour. It appears to be completely absorbed in both fasting and non-fasting states. Cerebrospinal fluid penetration is only 2 percent in dogs and monkeys; preliminary human data suggest some cerebrospinal fluid penetration. Patients with AIDS or ARC currently are being enrolled in phase I clinical trials. Side effects observed so far include peripheral neuropathy, a variety of rashes, fever, aphthous stomatitis, thrombocytopenia, lactic dehydrogenase elevation, and anemia (greater than 20-percent decrease in hemoglobin). Whether these toxicities limit this drug's usefulness remains to be determined.

Newer agents

Several novel anti-HIV agents also are under development. Ampligen is mismatched, double-stranded RNA that protects lymphoblastoid cells from HIV infection in vitro. Eleven patients with ARC or AIDS were given the drug in doses of 200 mg to 250 mg twice weekly for 12 to 16 weeks, with half the dose given subsequently as maintenance therapy. Skin test anergy returned for all patients, and lymphadenopathy was resolved in three of five patients. Virologic changes, including reduction in p24 antigen, were observed in nine of 11 patients. T4 cell numbers increased in three patients and were stable in the others. No patient showed side effects. One patient died following an episode of Pneumocystis carinii pneumonia after seven weeks of ampligen therapy. Continued experience with this agent will be necessary before any benefit can be concluded.

Castanospermine exerts an anti-HIV effect by altering the env glycoprotein of HIV and decreasing gp120 production, versus altering the T4 molecule. The drug appears to inhibit lymphocyte syncytium formation by the virus and therefore may be useful in slowing the depletion of T4 cells, which is thought to be possibly attributable to syncytium formation. Phosphate analogs of nucleosides inhibit HIV in vitro by preventing normal synthesis of viral DNA. Preclinical testing of these analogs is now under way.

Combinations of anti-retrovirals: Synergism/antagonism

Several combinations of antivirals have demonstrated additive, synergistic or antagonistic effects for inhibition of HIV. Studies suggest that combinations of drugs may have enhanced clinical efficacy and may inhibit HIV replication at better-tolerated levels and more easily achieved concentrations in vivo. Additionally, such combinations may prevent selection of drug-resistant HIV mutants. Presently, however, no evidence supports correlations between in-vitro synergy and enhanced clinical outcome.

The interactions between zidovudine and interferon and between zidovudine and the antiviral acyclovir have stimulated interest in HIV combination therapy. In vitro, both these drugs enhance zidovudine's inhibition of HIV. The mechanism of acyclovir-zidovudine synergism is unknown; however, because acyclovir is a well-tolerated drug with no hematologic toxicity, its use with zidovudine appears encouraging. Alpha interferon prevents release of infectious viruses and, hence, inhibits HIV at a different stage in the viral replication process than zidovudine. The AIDS Treatment Evaluation Unit program of the National Institutes of Health plans phase I trials with this combination. Additionally, lymphoblastoid interferon has been found to be synergistic with zidovudine in vitro.

Not all antivirals are additive or synergistic. This fact is illustrated by the in-vitro antagonistic effects between zidovudine and ribavirin. Ribavirin appears to increase deoxythymidine triphosphate levels which, in turn, cause feedback inhibition of thymidine kinase. This reduces phosphorylation of zidovudine to zidovudine-TP. These data also suggest ribavirin should not be used in vivo with zidovudine or similar derivatives except under investigational conditions. The clinical importance of the in-vitro antagonism of zidovudine and ribarivin requires clarification. On a more positive note, ribavirin has been shown to be synergistic in vitro with PFA.

Treating the HIV-infected patient with anti-retroviral agents: The options

There currently are several avenues through which an HIV-infected patient may receive anti-retroviral therapy. These include: FDA-approved agents, study protocols governed by the National Institutes of Health, and study protocols governed by the pharmaceutical industry.

Since zidovudine is the only FDA-approved agent, this option is limited to eligible patients. As of late September 1987, Retrovir™ distribution procedures were revised so that all physicians can prescribe zidovudine for eligible patients without special permission from Burroughs Wellcome Co. However, information is lacking on zidovudine's efficacy and safety in HIV-infected patients who do not fulfill FDA-approved criteria. We urge physicians not to prescribe zidovudine for persons who do not meet the package insert guidelines. The need is evident for controlled studies of persons in the earlier stages of HIV infection, and several such studies are under way. The benefits vs. risks of zidovudine in these patients are unknown.

Congress recently appropriated $30 million nationally—of which the Washington Department of Social and Health Services received approximately $354,000—to allow certain persons to receive zidovudine. Reimbursement for zidovudine is available for some low-income persons who lack Medicaid assistance, third-party medical insurance with prescription drug coverage, or income in excess of 185 percent of the national poverty level. To apply for support in Washington state, the prescribing physician and patient must complete an eligibility application form. This form, along with the name and address of the dispensing pharmacy, must be sent to the Washington Department of Social and Health Services, AIDS Prescription Drug Program, Mail Stop LP-13, Olympia, WA 98504. The AIDS Program staff will determine if the patient is eligible for full or partial payment. For further information, call the department's John Peppert or Joan Clark at 206-586-0426.

Prospects in antiretroviral chemotherapy for treatment of HIV infection

In November 1987 the National Institutes of Health reorganized 35 research centers (previously ATEUs and Clinical Study Groups) to form the AIDS Clinical Trials Group (ACTGs). Currently, many clinical trials are under way and numerous others are being planned. These include evaluation of two doses of zidovudine in the patients who have recovered from an episode of *Pneumocystis carinii* pneumonia; a placebo-controlled trial to evaluate zidovudine therapy in children with AIDS or ARC; antineoplastic-drug therapy, radiotherapy, and zidovudine therapy for high-grade lymphoma in patients at risk for AIDS; and dideoxycytidine pharmacokinetics in HIV-infected patients. Other trials include a multicenter dose-finding study of dideoxycytidine in the treatment of advanced ARC; zidovudine and human interferon in the treatment of AIDS-associated Kaposi's sarcoma; evaluation of zidovudine therapy in patients with hemophilia; a multicenter trial to evaluate the long-term safety and patient tolerance of zidovudine for the treatment of HIV infections in persons with AIDS and advanced ARC; safety and efficacy of zidovudine for asymptomatic HIV-infected patients. A number of other investigations with zidovudine are under way to assess potential drug interactions (e.g., with ganciclovir, trimethoprim-sulfamethoxazole, pentamidine). The collaborative efforts of the ACTGs should expedite large, multicenter, controlled clinical trials with antiretroviral agents and speed the search for a cure.

Summary

Antivirals might attack any of several potential targets to inhibit HIV replication and/or to eradicate the latent form in infected cells. Antivirals could interfere with the cell receptor for HIV; prevent uncoating; inhibit reverse transcriptase; prevent integration/post-transcription processing; or inhibit assembly or release. Most agents developed thus far inhibit HIV's reverse transcriptase. Agents with *in-vitro* activity against HIV include zidovudine, dideoxycytidine, ammonium 21-tungsto-9-antimoniate (HPA-23), ribavirin, and phosphonoformate (PFA, Foscarnet™). Ultimately, combinations of agents may be employed. However, the use of concomitant anti-HIV agents requires careful evaluation.

To date, zidovudine is the only FDA-approved agent that appears to be a clinically effective anti-retroviral agent. Zidovudine use currently is restricted to patients who have overt AIDS, or symptomatic ARC with less than 200 circulating T4 cells/mm3. Zidovudine toxicities—including neutropenia and anemia—are significant. Careful monitoring of hematologic parameters is essential when using zidovudine, and dose reduction and occasional discontinuance of zidovudine may be necessary. Co-administration of other drugs, such as acetaminophen, should be avoided or done with utmost caution. Because zidovudine is not a cure for HIV infection and because HIV appears to be a lifelong infection requiring chronic treatment, numerous studies are under way with many other anti-HIV agents. Studies are also under way to see if zidovudine can be used earlier in the course of HIV infection. While the search for more efficacious and less toxic treatments continues, zidovudine's short-term development provides hope that further progress in this area will continue at its present rapid pace.

Additional Reading

Fischl, M.A., Richman, D.D., Grieco, M.H., Gottlieb, M.S., Volberding, P.A. *et al.* 1986. The efficacy of azidothymidine (AZT) in the treatment of patients with AIDS and AIDS-related complex. *N Engl J Med* 317:185-191.

Francis, D.P., Petricciani, J.C. 1985. The prospects for and pathways toward a vaccine for AIDS (special article). *N Engl J Med* 313:1586-1590.

Hirsch, M., Kaplan, J.C. 1987. Treatment of human immunodeficiency virus infections (minireview). *Antimicrob Agents and Chemother* 31:839-844.

Mitsuya, H., Broder, S. 1987. Strategies for antiviral therapy in AIDS (review article). *Nature* 325:773-778.

Richman, D.D., Fischl, M.A., Grieco, M.H., Gottlieb, M.S., Volberding, P.A., Laskin, O.L., Leedom, J.M. *et al.* 1987. The toxicity of azidothymidine (AZT) in the treatment of patients with AIDS and AIDS-related complex. *N Engl J Med* 317:192-197.

Vogt, M., Hirsch, M.S. 1986. Prospects for the prevention and therapy of infections with the human immunodeficiency virus (serial features). *Reviews of Infectious Diseases* 8:991-1000.

Table V AIDS Clinical Trial Groups

Albert Einstein College of Medicine (New York City) Dr. Ruy Soeiro (212) 430–2371	Cornell University Medical College (New York City) Dr. Henry Murray (212) 472–6800	Massachusetts Medical School, University of (Worcester) Dr. Neil Blacklow (617) 856–3158	Norris Cancer Hospital and Research Institute (Los Angeles) Dr. Alexandra Levine (213) 224–6668	San Francisco General Hospital Dr. John Mills (415) 821–8666
Bellevue Hospital (New York City) Dr. Fred T. Valentine (212) 340–6401	Duke University Medical Center (Durham, North Carolina) Dr. Dani P. Bolognesi (919) 684–3103	Memorial Hospital for Cancer and Allied Diseases (NYC) Dr. Donald Armstrong (212) 794–7809	Northwestern University Medical School (Chicago, Illinois) Dr. John Phair (312) 908–8196	Southern California, University of (Los Angeles) Dr. John Leedom (213) 226–7504
California, University of (Los Angeles) Dr. David Golde (213) 825–1301	George Washington Univ. Medical Ctr. (Washington, D.C.) Dr. Richard Schulof (202) 994–8395	Miami, University of (FLA) Dr. Margaret A. Fischl (305) 549–7416	North Carolina, University of (Chapel Hill) Dr. Stanley Lemon (919) 966–2536	Stanford University (Palo Alto) Dr. Thomas C. Merigan (415) 725–3929
California, University of (San Diego) Dr. Stephen A. Spector (619) 294–6447	Harvard University Massachusetts General Hosp. (Boston) Dr. Martin Hirsch (617) 726–3815	Milton S. Hershey Medical Ctr. (Hershey, Pennsylvania) Dr. M. Eyster (717) 531–8399	Ohio State University Medical Center (Columbus) Dr. Robert Fass (614) 293–8732	State University of New York at Stony Brook Dr. Roy Steigbigel (516) 444–1660
Children's Hospital Corporation (Boston) Dr. Kenneth McIntosh (617) 735–7621	Indiana University School of Medicine (Indianapolis) Dr. Robert Jones (317) 274–8115	Minnesota, University of (Minneapolis) Dr. Henry H. Balfour, Jr. (612) 626–5670	Pittsburgh, University of Dr. Monto Ho (412) 624–2692	Tulane University Medical Center (New Orleans, Louisiana) Dr. Newton E. Hyslop, Jr. (504) 587–7316
Cincinnati, University of (Cincinnati) Dr. Peter Frame (513) 872–4704	Johns Hopkins Hospital (Baltimore, Maryland) Dr. John G. Bartlett (301) 955–3150	New Jersey Medical School (Newark, NJ) Dr. Edward Connor (201) 268–8464	Rochester, University of (New York) Dr. Raphael Dolin (716) 275–5770	Washington, University of (Seattle) Dr. Lawrence Corey (206) 223–3293
Cleveland, University Hospitals of (Cleveland) Dr. Michael Lederman (216) 844–3245	Mt. Sinai School of Medicine (New York City) Dr. Henry S. Sacks (212) 650–7856	University of Medicine and Dentistry of New Jersey (New Brunswick, NJ) Dr. David Gocke (201) 937–7710	St. Lukes/Roosevelt Hospital Med. Ctr. (New York City) Dr. Michael Grieco (212) 554–7194	Washington University School of Medicine (St. Louis, MO) Dr. Lee Ratner (314) 362–8836

Psychosocial Aspects of AIDS

by Terence C. Gayle, M.D., Lewayne D. Gilchrist, Ph.D., and Heather Andersen, R.N., M.N.

Primary care physicians will be increasingly involved in the direct care of patients with human immunodeficiency virus (HIV) disorders ranging from asymptomatic HIV-antibody seropositivity to acquired immunodeficiency syndrome (AIDS). The physical conditions of such patients are inextricably bound to their individual psychological processes, as well as to the reactions of the people around them. Physicians must recognize the psychosocial component of suffering and how psychological and social issues contribute to the disease process and provision of care. Awareness of these issues is essential to the integrity of the physician-patient relationship and to fulfillment of the oldest and most important goal of the profession—to relieve suffering, regardless of the chances for cure. Accomplishing this goal requires frank discussion about fears surrounding the disease, treatment options, risk reduction, and also referral to a variety of mental health and social service resources when appropriate.

At least three realities complicate physicians' ability to care for patients with AIDS-related diseases. The first is our constantly changing understanding of the pathophysiology of HIV infection. AIDS-related diseases are varied and sometimes hard to identify, and their course is often unpredictable. Prognosis is often uncertain. Statistics regarding prevalence, prognosis, and modes of transmission may not answer the questions and concerns of an individual patient.

The second reality is that persons at highest risk for AIDS are members of stigmatized social groups. Identifying a patient's actual risk status requires taking a careful history of sexual behavior and patterns of intravenous (IV) drug use. Physicians usually have little training in this area and may be reluctant to question patients directly on these topics.

The third reality is the frequent necessity to coordinate aspects of care for HIV-infected patients with other care providers in the community. Out-of-hospital care for debilitated AIDS and AIDS-related complex (ARC) patients may require the cooperation of at least one social service

agency. The crushing emotional reactions of many patients, plus the necessity to help patients make lasting changes in their sexual behavior, may require referral to psychiatrists and other mental health professionals. Many physicians are unaware of such resources in their communities, and many communities lack such resources altogether.

In this article we illustrate psychosocial issues as they relate to five groups. The first three groups include people with AIDS; people with ARC (including persistent generalized lymphadenopathy), and asymptomatic seropositive people. The other two groups include the worried well: high-risk group members who thus far are seronegative; and low-risk group members who are seronegative but are concerned about their health. Patients in each of these groups face clinically relevant psychological, social and behavioral issues.

Issues related to the diagnosis of AIDS

In many ways, reactions to AIDS are similar to those seen in cancer and other life-threatening illnesses. We can examine the process of coping with catastrophic illness in a framework of three phases of adaptation. The process begins with initial awareness of the threat, proceeds through a transitional period of actively integrating limitations into daily life, and usually ends in a new state of psychic equilibrium marked by an acceptance of the imposed limitations.

The notion of stages of adaptation is offered here as a general guideline only. Actual movement through these phases is often neither linear nor orderly. Rather than progressing to an ultimate resolution, a person recycles through the set of phases with each subsequent adverse event—such as a decline in health status. This framework is relevant to clinical care because it can help the clinician make an optimal match between an intervention and the patient's stage of adaptation.

Persons newly diagnosed with AIDS experience an initial crisis marked by waves of extreme anxiety that alternate between denial and a feeling of emotional numbness. The initial shock of diagnosis may be less intense in persons who already suspect they have AIDS because of a recent gradual decline in health status associated with ARC. In this first phase, persons with AIDS may be too overwhelmed to remember many details of medical information

presented. The best therapeutic stance is to provide emotional support, answer repeated questions as honestly as possible without taking away hope,[1] and acknowledge that intense emotions are part of a normal stress response syndrome. The initial crisis phase can last from days to several weeks and corresponds roughly to the period of the first hospitalization or the first few weeks after the diagnosis of Kaposi's sarcoma on an outpatient basis.

Shortly after the diagnosis is confirmed, patients are confronted with a barrage of questions and decisions, such as whom to inform, who else may be at risk, what to tell employers, how to handle changes in finances and home arrangements, and how to evaluate treatment options. In this stage, persons with AIDS will benefit from a crisis-intervention approach that reinforces previous psychological strengths and breaks the wall of difficult problems into smaller pieces that can be managed one at a time. The patient needs to know that hasty decisions are not necessary and that time is available to deal with most of these issues.

A certain amount of denial is adaptive in the early stages. However, too strong a persistent denial of the diagnosis and its implications can lead to non-compliance with medical care or failure to make necessary practical decisions. Because social support is so critical, involvement of the person's significant other or closest friend in discussions and plans is an essential means of enhancing coping.

After the initial crisis resolves, AIDS patients enter a middle or transitional phase. During this period, the person with AIDS struggles with two tasks: coping with the practical problems of daily living in the face of increasing disability, and anticipatory grieving over future losses. Existential issues related to the meaning of one's life, along with fears of death and dying, become paramount. AIDS is particularly isolating, since it is associated with such highly politically and emotionally charged issues as homosexuality, presumed sexual promiscuity, drug use, fear of contagion, and death. Fear of loneliness and abandonment can be eased by scheduling regular follow-up appointments with a consistent primary care physician, referring persons to AIDS support groups or individual counselors, and linking them with volunteer "buddies" or companions such as those in the Seattle SHANTI organization (see "The Public Health Response to AIDS" on page 10). Physical contact—a massage or even an empathetic hand on the shoulder—

Dr. Gayle is a Veterans Administration Fellow in the Robert Wood Johnson Clinical Scholars Program at the University of Washington and is a UW acting instructor of psychiatry and behavioral sciences. Dr. Gilchrist is a research associate professor in the UW School of Social Work. Ms. Andersen is a lecturer in the UW School of Social Work and the UW School of Nursing.

---

1 An example of an honest yet supportive statement to a patient with newly diagnosed Kaposi's sarcoma might be: "You have Kaposi's sarcoma. So far, the average life expectancy for someone with KS is about two years, but some people have had KS for several years and are still living productive lives. Research on AIDS antiviral drugs and other treatment is moving quickly. With good nutrition, stress management, rest, regular exercise, and avoidance of new infections, you could help keep the virus from gaining an even bigger foothold and from progressing as rapidly."

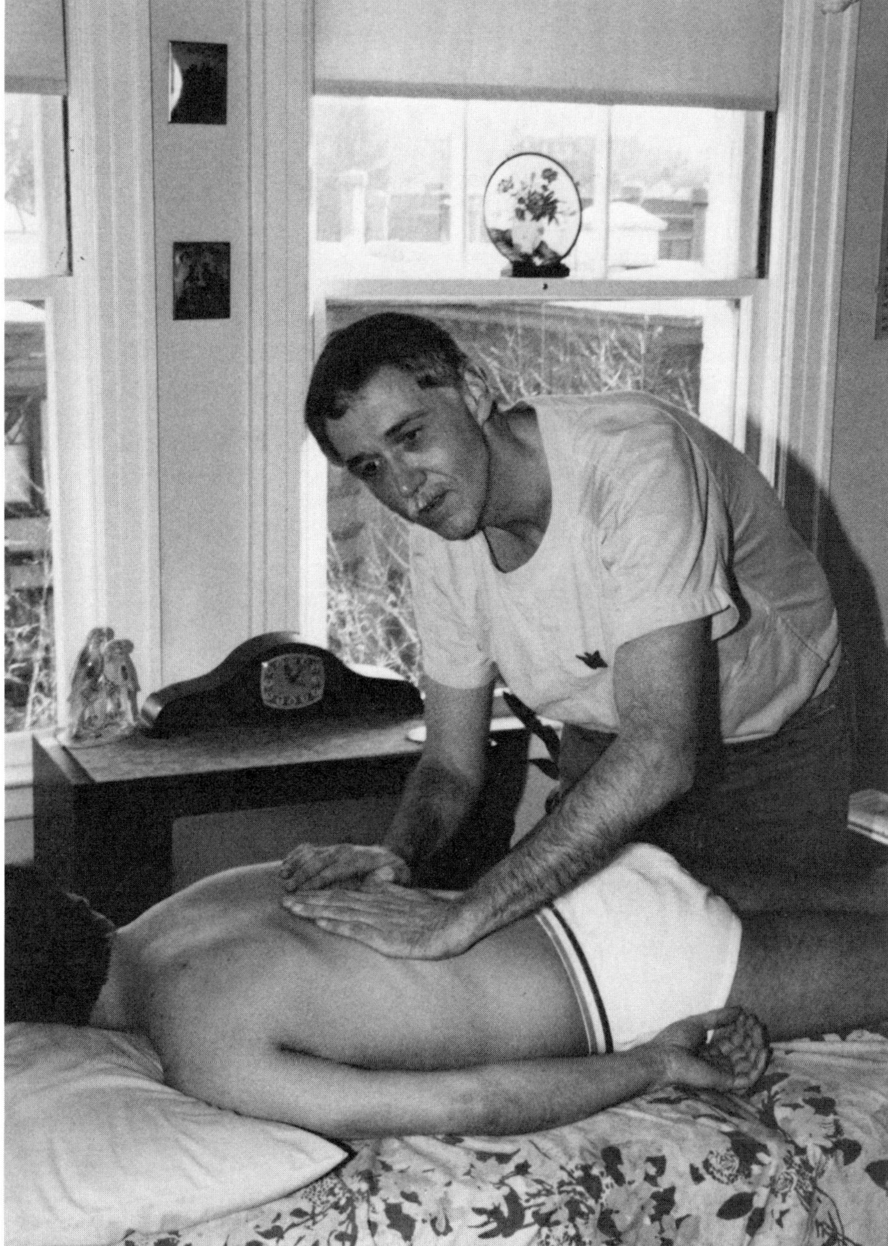

FIGURE 1. Seattle massage therapist Bob Fuller donates his time to work with AIDS patients.

provides a sense of comfort and cuts through feelings of isolation and loneliness (Figure 1). Since many persons with AIDS have known others who died of AIDS, their fears of pain and suffering are realistic. Gruesome expectations may be ameliorated by early discussion of palliative treatment options for pain and other symptoms. To sustain hope and to counter fears of dependency and loss of control, it is vital that the person retain as much autonomy as is permitted by his physical condition. Patients need to participate as equal partners in making all treatment decisions.

Home care is more humane than prolonged hospitalization and is perhaps a more cost-effective alternative. As disability increases, chore care services can help keep a person in the home longer. If a person's sense of identity is closely bound to a job, then encouragement to return to the job or to participate in volunteer work can help fend off the fear of loss of identity. The fear of disfigurement in young people concerned about body image can often be lessened by empathic statements that reinforce the intrinsic worth and good of the person regardless of emaciation or Kaposi's sarcoma lesions.

Persons with AIDS describe being on an emotional roller-coaster in response to changes brought on by the disease process. A resurgence of hopelessness is most likely to occur at the time of treatment failure or subsequent re-hospitalization. The personal meaning of the disease for the AIDS patient is often the source of much suffering. Rumination over the question "Why me?" frequently leads to guilt about sexual orientation, past sexual partners, or other lifestyle factors. We cannot overemphasize the importance of helping alleviate this guilt to reduce the total burden of suffering.

Persons with AIDS need to be reminded that they have AIDS not because of who they are but because they are infected with the causative virus.

Most persons with AIDS will admit to thoughts about suicide. Sometimes the idea seems to represent a somewhat comforting symbol of self-determination and destiny in the face of so much that is uncontrollable. Negotiable environmental changes—for example, housing, assistance and companionship—and counseling about relationship problems can sometimes dramatically reduce suicidal intent. The incidence of suicide in AIDS patients is not well-defined, but the experience of the gay community on the West Coast suggests that suicide is relatively infrequent.

The recent availability of zidovudine (formerly known as azidothymidine or AZT) has provided a source of hope for persons with AIDS but also may create additional complexities for patients trying to make decisions about treatment and the future. They must weigh the benefits of prolonged life against zidovudine's high cost and the possibility of drug intolerance or the need for frequent transfusions. One of zidovudine's most gratifying benefits may be its ability to reverse or at least halt the AIDS dementia syndrome.

Persons with AIDS often experience dramatic realignments of the spiritual and philosophical aspects of their lives. The adaptive focus on the quality of their remaining time may result in a new, positive spirit that can have a powerful effect on their friends and caregivers.

One issue that sometimes surfaces is the compatibility of traditional medical care with alternative treatments. A patient's active search for alternatives can be an important part of coping and should not be immediately discouraged. Patient-physician agreements on concurrent strategies are possible whereby the physician is informed of alternative treatments and tells the patient about potential harm.

A significant proportion of patients suffer the additional burden of AIDS dementia complex, major depression, and other psychiatric disorders associated with medical illness (see "Clinical Manifestations and Approach to Management of HIV Infection and AIDS," page 27). In particular, major depression is suggested by prolonged loss of self-esteem, unremitting guilt, and the inability to experience pleasure in anything. Because of the high probability of eventual cognitive dysfunction, persons with AIDS should be strongly encouraged to take an active part in getting their affairs in order as early as possible after diagnosis. Such business includes completing wills, designating durable power of attorney, and making funeral arrangements. These activities promote a sense of personal control. Code status should be determined within the first 72 hours of each hospitalization in accordance with the patient's wishes.

The terminal phase occupies the final days or weeks before death. During this time, the AIDS patient turns inward and retreats from the world. Since family and loved ones may feel rejected, it is helpful to reinterpret this for them as part of the natural death cycle, thus giving the patient permission to withdraw. The dying person may feel the need to complete unfinished personal business with loved ones. The caregiver's principal goal is to facilitate a death that is as free of pain and isolation as possible. During all phases, persons with AIDS are especially subject to social isolation imposed by some hospital infection control procedures and the avoidance behaviors of some health care workers. Such isolation can be lessened by explaining any necessary precautions to the patient and by acknowledging and confronting our own fears of AIDS and our attitudes toward members of high-risk groups.

John's case example points out one of the most important aspects of care for AIDS patients: the need for a multidisciplinary team approach. Caring for persons with AIDS is difficult even with access to the best resources. No one primary care clinician could possibly provide all the facets of care required. We strongly urge case management with orchestration of a variety of services as a means of providing efficient and quality care and preventing provider burnout.

C A S E   1

AIDS

John is 32 years old, gay and white. He was diagnosed as having ARC a year before his first episode of *Pneumocystis carinii* pneumonia (PCP). His local support system includes a lover of three years and several friends. He was successfully employed as a bookkeeper at an insurance company, but had to quit the job six months ago because of difficulties with routine arithmetic. The problem was caused by slow but progressive cognitive dysfunction.

Acute Crisis Phase:
—John's lover is included in discussions of a treatment plan.

—John's physician asks if John wants his parents to know and if they know he is gay.

—John is referred to Seattle SHANTI so he can establish a relationship with a volunteer before discharge.

Transitional Phase:
—John's physician schedules biweekly follow-up appointments, refers John to a weekly AIDS support group, and refers John and his lover to a therapist for couples counseling around interpersonal conflicts resulting from the strain of AIDS.

—With the help of the Northwest AIDS Foundation and a group of volunteer lawyers who work with AIDS patients, John completes his will and arranges for his lover to have durable power of attorney if John becomes mentally incapacitated.

—John decides he does not want to be intubated if he has another episode of PCP.

—When John begins to appear depressed, withdraws socially and has more memory complaints, he is referred to a psychiatrist who diagnoses major depression and begins antidepressant treatment. The depression improves, but the cognitive dysfunction worsens.

—The psychiatrist has signs placed around John's house ("Turn off the stove") as memory aids.

—As John develops motor problems that limit ambulation, a chore care worker comes in to help with cleaning, cooking and bathing.

—John's lover is referred to a support group for partners and family of AIDS patients to vent his grief over John's declining health.

Terminal Phase:
—During the final hospitalization, John's physician and social worker conduct a family conference that includes John's parents and lover. They sort out individual responsibilities that make all parties feel useful.

—John dies, having completed unfinished business with his family and in the company of his lover.

—Memorial services are conducted according to John's wishes.

Issues related to ARC diagnosis

Research has consistently indicated that ARC patients experience higher overall levels of emotional distress than AIDS patients. Anxiety is the most prevalent mood disturbance. This is not surprising if one realizes that ARC patients live in a purgatory of uncertainty regarding prognosis. Prolonged anxiety may eventually give way to depression. Many ARC patients are keenly interested in their doctor's opinions of ways to prevent progression to AIDS, such as diet, vitamin use, and other possible preventions. One way to deal with the uncertainty is to shift perspective from concern about eventual death to living more in the present. Some persons with ARC undergo the same philosophical and spiritual development as those with AIDS. Relaxation training and positive imagery are effective in reducing anxiety and should be tried before prescribing benzodiazepines, unless the anxiety is functionally disabling.

Because of the imposed isolation and the relative lack of focused resources for persons with ARC, helping them find a support system is one of the best things a physician can do. They can benefit greatly from participation in support groups. Referral for couple counseling is indicated when ARC disrupts patients' interpersonal relationships or causes communication problems.

One should keep in mind that ARC patients also have an increased risk of developing such neuropsychiatric problems as cognitive dysfunction and major depression. In Case 1, John showed signs of an insidious dementia that led to work impairment well before the AIDS diagnosis was confirmed.

Issues related to seropositive diagnosis

For many people, confirmation of their seropositive status through the antibody test comes as a surprise even when they appear intellectually prepared for that possibility. Such confirmation can be acutely distressing (see Case 2). Irrefutable proof of infection can quite suddenly bring with it the lifelong specter of disability, disease, lost or irreparably changed sexual expression, and death—all of which young, physically well persons are ill-prepared to confront.

C A S E   2

Seropositive diagnosis

Roy, a 29-year-old gay man, recently ended a three-year relationship when his partner, Mark, left for a new job in a distant city. Roy and Mark had a mutually monogamous relationship. Although he and Mark had never used condoms, Roy had never worried about HIV infection or AIDS. Realizing that he is anxious about re-entering the dating scene and managing new sexual relationships, he decides somewhat impulsively to be tested for HIV antibodies. Disclosing his verified negative status to potential partners will be advantageous, he thinks, and his seronegativity will give him an incentive to stick with safer sex and other health-affirming practices.

Since Roy belongs to a high-risk group, he has no trouble being tested. He gives no real thought to the possibility that he might be seropositive. News of his seropositive status devastates him. He subsequently realizes that, although he knew that he and Mark had had a mutually monogamous relationship, he knows very little about Mark's life and sexual partners before they met.

Acute Crisis Phase:
—Give Roy time to absorb the news and to ventilate anger and other negative feelings.

—Do not attempt complex problem-solving or clinical instruction during the period of maximum emotional upset.

—Reassure Roy, if necessary, that he will not spread infection through casual contact with friends.

—Schedule a follow-up visit in a few days.

Acceptance Phase:
—Give Roy safe sex guidelines and discuss any problems he foresees in putting the guidelines into practice.

—Refer him to a support group for seropositive men.

—If necessary, plan with Roy how and when he will tell Mark about his HIV status and how Roy can advise Mark to be tested.

—If needed, refer Roy to a psychotherapist for help with anger at his ex-partner and with changing to safe sex.

—Advise Roy regarding nutrition and infection avoidance.

Following confirmation of seropositive status, most patients want to know their chances of developing ARC or AIDS. The data from recent longitudinal studies of seropositive gay men are sobering. Twenty percent to 35 percent of seropositive men developed AIDS over six to eight years. An additional 30 to 35 percent developed symptoms of ARC (such as persistent generalized lymphadenopathy and oral thrush) over the same period. Currently, we have little concrete information about the characteristics that differentiate those who develop full immune deficiency from those who do not. The gravity of the possibility of AIDS, coupled with the uncertainty of the prognosis, can lead to frustration for both physician and patient. Many seropositive patients want advice about diet, exercise, and other health-affirming activities to help them feel more in control of their health. Many want explicit information about how modes of virus transmission may affect their typical activities. They ask such questions as: "What kinds of casual contact are safe? Can I kiss my mother without worrying that I will harm her? How much at risk is my partner? Can I ever have sex again?"

Table I outlines accepted prevention guidelines. Physicians may be called upon to translate these general guidelines into the realities of everyday behavior in clear, unmistakable terms. Although transmission prevention guidelines seem clear, they can be extraordinarily difficult to put into practice. For example, intellectual commitment to using condoms at every sexual encounter can quickly break down when negotiating condom use with a partner one doesn't want to alienate, or when judgment is impaired by alcohol or recreational drugs. Among some groups of IV drug abusers, a culture of sharing "works" (needles) exists that is virtually impossible to avoid without dissociating from the group entirely. If the group provides a person's only social support, such dissociation may be extremely difficult. Where compliance with transmission prevention guidelines may be especially difficult, it may be very helpful to refer the patient to a psychiatrist, psychologist, social worker, or other behavioral specialist.

Research on compliance suggests that a simple and effective way to assess probable compliance is to ask the patient in a nonjudgmental way, "Do you think you will be able to use a condom every time you have intercourse, or do you think you will probably not be able to arrange this?" If the patient anticipates trouble, ask "Would you like to be referred for counseling to teach you how to do this?" Local health departments in larger cities can help with referral for such counseling (see information sources listed on the back cover).

Newly diagnosed seropositive patients usually have many concerns about the con-

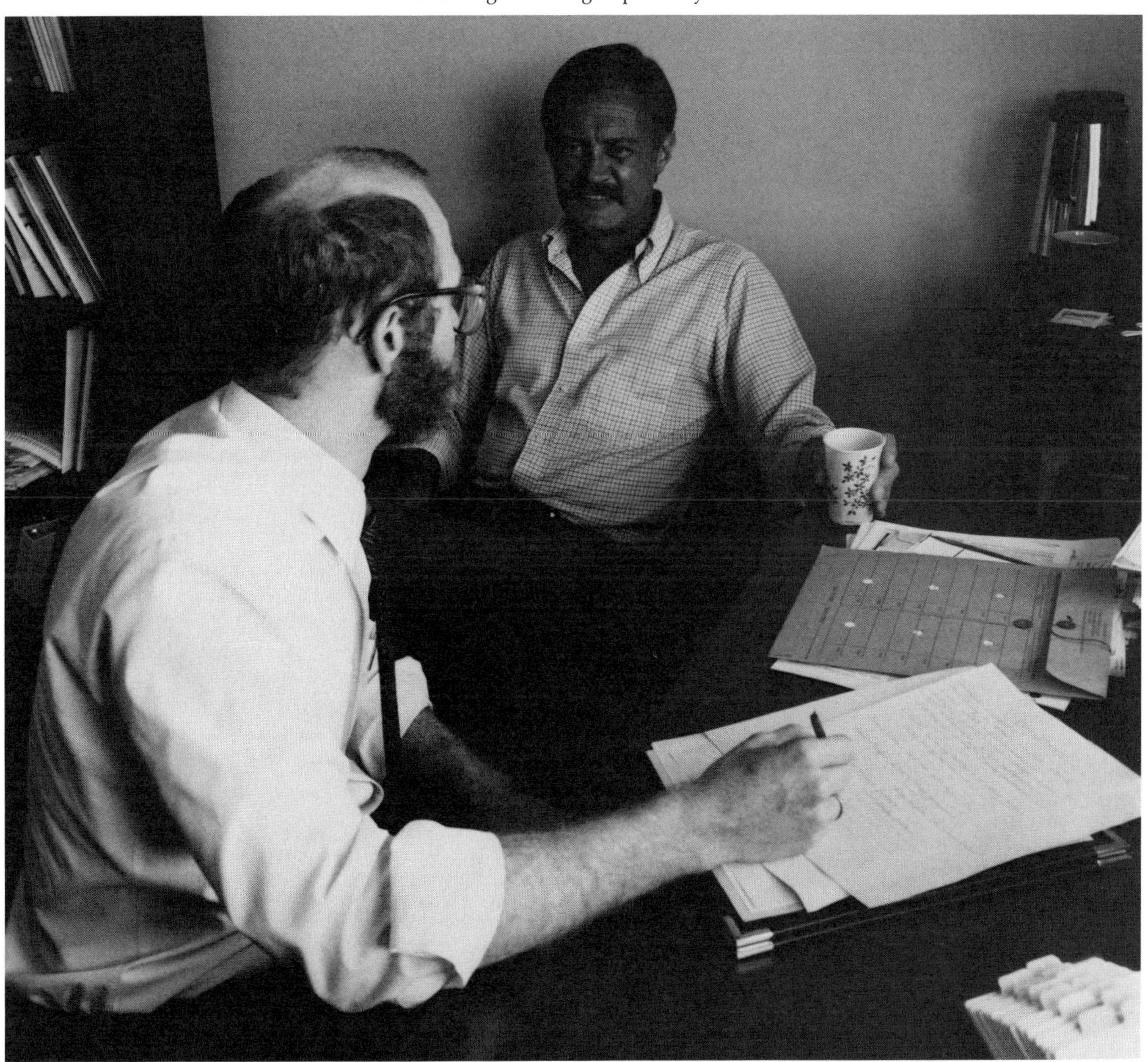

FIGURE 2. Dick Fusco (right), diagnosed as having AIDS-related complex (ARC) in 1984, meets with Dr. Terence Gayle (left) twice a month for psychotherapy to discuss such complications as depression, concentration problems and lack of energy.

fidentiality of their test results. Patients may have serious and realistic worries that they will lose their jobs or health insurance if their status is disclosed to an employer or an insurer. Physicians, clinics and hospitals treating HIV-infected patients will need to consider how they will deal with these important confidentiality issues. Legal counsel regarding such matters may be helpful.

Seropositive patients in sexual relationships need to inform their partners of their HIV-positive status. Physicians can help patients plan this disclosure and should strongly suggest that patients' partners voluntarily take the antibody test and receive counseling about infection control. A disturbing ethical dilemma arises when a physician knows that a seropositive patient is continuing unprotected, high-risk sexual activities with an uninformed partner. In this instance, the duty to warn those at risk is at odds with the professional commitment to confidentiality. All those who treat seropositive patients should examine their own values and consider what actions they would take if confronted with this dilemma. The Centers for Disease Control advocates the use of confidential procedures for partner notification when an HIV-infected person is unwilling to notify his or her partner or if it cannot be assured that the partner will seek counseling.

Issues related to seronegative diagnosis: The worried well

Patients in this diagnostic category fall into two groups: those whose past or current behavior places them at high, real risk of infection; and those whose past and current behavior makes infection unlikely or highly improbable. Physicians should be knowledgeable about the pros and cons of the antibody test or be able to refer patients to someone who is. To assess advisability of testing an individual patient, physicians should do a history thorough enough to realistically assess the patient's risk status. Many health care providers do not routinely ask patients about sexual behavior or about drug use and possible needle sharing. If physicians assume a patient's risk status without taking a structured history focused on specific high-risk behavior, they can misjudge the patient's true vulnerability.

C A S E 3

Seronegative, high risk of infection

Stan, age 29, has been married for four years and has a satisfying sexual relationship with his wife. Stan's job requires extensive travel. During his travels—without his wife's knowledge—Stan has unprotected anal intercourse with men he meets in gay bars. Although Stan knows he may be risking infection and may be placing his wife at risk as well, he has not considered antibody testing. He feels certain that if his wife or his employer knew of his homosexual activities, he would lose everything.

Table I Guidelines for Prevention of HIV Infection

To stop sexual transmission:

Safe:

—sexual abstinence

—non-insertive sexual relations: hugging, kissing (if no oral lesions present), genital manipulation (if no skin lesions present)

—social (dry) kissing

—body-to-body rubbing ("frottage")

—fantasy

Possibly Safe:

—insertive sexual relations (anal and vaginal) with proper use of condoms

—french kissing (wet)

—exchange of body fluids, external only (for example, skin contact with urine or saliva)

—fellatio but stopping before climax

—cunnilingus (mouth on vulva or clitoris)

Not safe:

—rimming (touching anus with tongue)

—fisting (inserting fingers or hands in rectum)

—any contact involving blood

—sharing insertive sex toys

—semen or urine in mouth

—insertive sexual intercourse (vaginal or anal) without a condom

To stop needle-borne transmission:
Do not use unsterile needles or share needles or syringes.

To stop perinatal transmission:
Be tested for antibodies; if you are positive, do not become pregnant.

During a routine physical exam, Stan casually remarks that AIDS affects only "flaming queers." His physician says that HIV infection occurs because of particular behavior regardless of sexual orientation. Stan's distressed reaction leads his physician to ask pointed questions about past, possibly high-risk behavior. Stan and his physician agree that he should be tested for HIV antibodies.

Stan's test shows him to be seronegative. He tells his physician that he wants to stay that way but isn't sure he can control his sexual behavior.

—Listen carefully for underlying true concerns.

—Obtain a sexual history complete enough to assess Stan's real risk status.

—Allay Stan's fears regarding the confidentiality of antibody test results.

—Assess Stan's ability to cope with possible confirmation of seropositive status. Make sure he fully understands the nature of the test and its consequences, or refer him to someone who can do this pre-test counseling.

—Do an antibody test or refer Stan for testing. Advise him to have a second test in two to three months to avoid the possibility that he has been infected but hasn't yet developed antibodies.

—Give Stan clear guidelines on safe sex practices.

—Provide him with references for counseling or mental health resources to help him achieve lasting behavior change to reduce his risk of infection.

Stan's reasonably satisfactory relationship with his wife could lead to the assumption of exclusive heterosexuality and, therefore, low-risk status. A better practice is to inquire directly whether the patient has engaged in unprotected anal intercourse since 1978, especially as a passive recipient, or has shared an IV needle or syringe since 1978. Most patients who have engaged in high-risk behavior will not volunteer this information until asked directly in a nonjudgmental manner. Research has shown that less than one-third of homosexual patients disclose their sexual orientation to their physician unless queried directly in the context of AIDS risk assessment. Chances are 3 percent to 5 percent that Stan may be infected despite being seronegative, but simply has not had time to develop detectable antibodies. Physicians may wish to recommend a second test approximately six months later for seronegative patients who are members of high-risk groups.

Patients like Stan may benefit from counseling to help them change long-standing behavior that puts them at risk for infection. Making changes in behavior patterns is not easy; changing sexual behavior in particular is quite difficult. Physicians should have available a list of referral resources—local self-help groups or psychiatrists and other mental health professionals in private practice, counseling and mental health agencies—to help the patient achieve lasting, protective behavior change.

Finally, some patients' psychological makeup leads to irrational fears that they have or will get AIDS. Discomfort with sexuality in general, guilt over perceived past indiscretions, and a host of other psychological reasons can lead to acute worry or even panic among patients who have little real risk of infection. Medical personnel can use their authority and credibility to reassure such patients that the risk of HIV infection is negligible and that testing is unnecessary. If reassurance proves insufficient, referral for counseling and mental health care—perhaps in addition to serologic testing—may alleviate patients' very real anguish.

The opinions, conclusions and proposals in this article are those of the authors and may not represent the views of the Robert Wood Johnson Foundation or the Veterans Administration.

Additional Reading

Cohen, M.A., and Weisman, H.W. 1986. A biopsychosocial approach to AIDS. *Psychosomatics* 27:245-249.

Faulstich, M.E. 1987. Psychiatric aspects of AIDS. *Am J Psychiatry* 144:551-556.

Holland, J. C., and Tross, S. 1985. The psychosocial and neuropsychiatric sequelae of the acquired immunodeficiency syndrome and related disorders. *Ann Intern Med* 103:760-764.

McKusick, L., Horstman, W., Abrams, D., and Coates, T.J. 1986. The psychological impact of AIDS on primary care physicians. *West J Med* 144:751-752.

Nichols, S.E. 1985. Psychosocial reactions of persons with the acquired immunodeficiency syndrome. *Ann Intern Med* 103:765-767.

Perry, S., and Jacobsen, P. 1986. Neuropsychiatric manifestations of AIDS-spectrum disorders. *Hosp Community Psychiatry* 37:135-142.

Wolcott, D. L., Namir, S., Fawzy, F., *et al.* 1986. Illness concerns, attitudes towards homosexuality, and social support in gay men with AIDS. *Gen Hosp Psychiatry* 8:395-403.

The Duty to Treat Patients with AIDS

by Albert R. Jonsen, Ph.D.

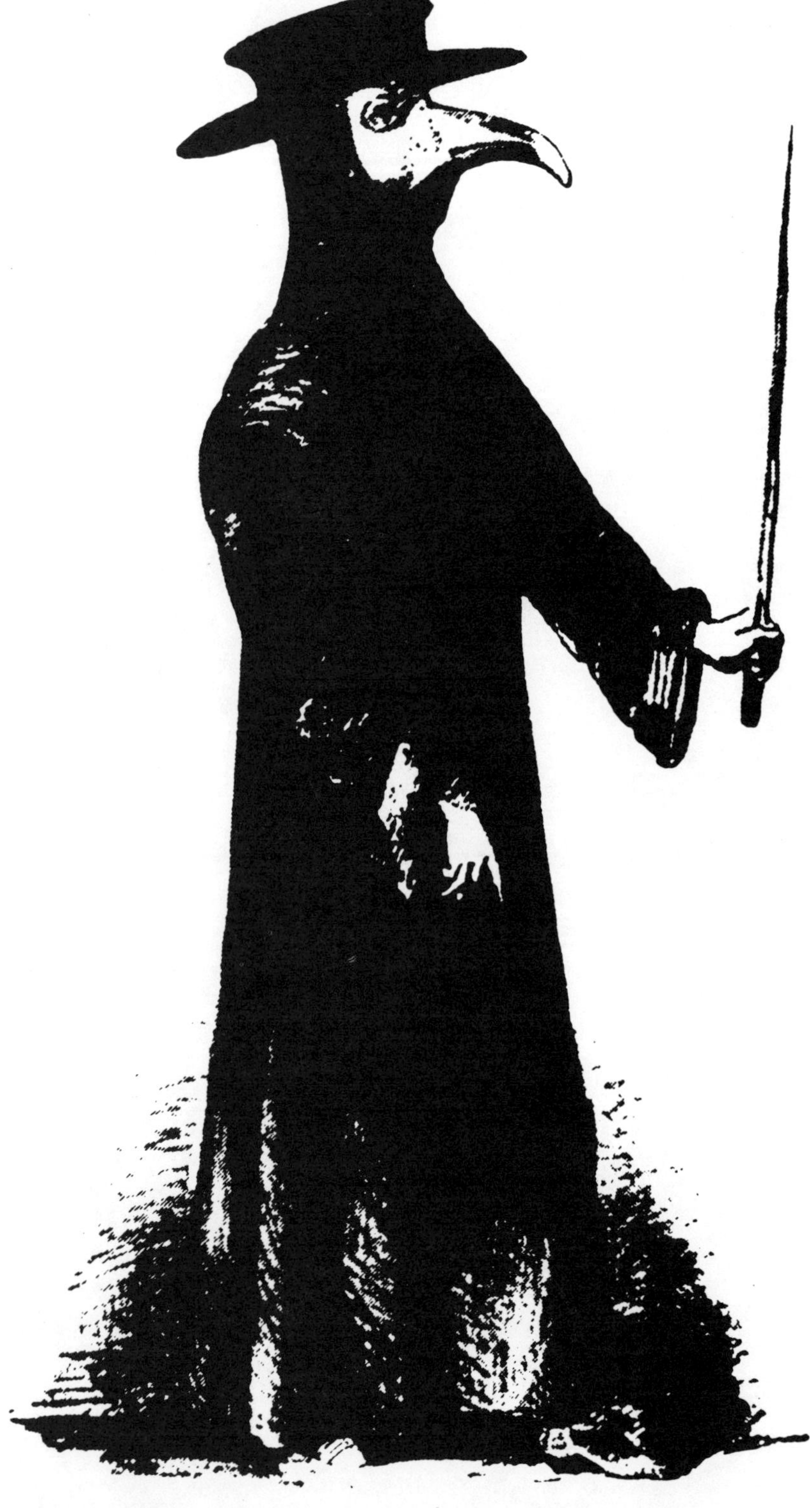

This physician is dressed in the garb worn during the bubonic plague epidemics in Italy in the 1600s. The heavy cloak functioned as a "body glove" to ward off the alleged atmospheric poisons believed to spread plague. Because people also believed such poisons leaked through the skin and were exhaled in breath, the spice-filled beak was relied upon as an air purifier and the wooden stick made it possible to take a pulse without touch.

Is it ethically permissible for a physician to refuse to treat a patient with acquired immunodeficiency syndrome (AIDS) or who has positive test results for human immunodeficiency virus (HIV) antibody?

The Principles of Ethics of the American Medical Association state that a physician may choose those whom he or she wishes to serve. American law does not require physicians to provide services to any particular patient, unless some special relationship already exists. Thus, it would appear that no physician has either a professional or a legal obligation to treat an AIDS patient.

However, there is more to ethics than the official statements of professional associations and the minimal obligations of the law. The role of the physician in our culture has always been identified with a willingness to serve those in need even at cost to self. This has been an important ingredient in the positive reputation of medicine and of physicians.

Does this reputation amount to an ethical principle? If it does, how strictly must it be observed? Are there circumstances in which a physician may refuse to respond to a person's need without being considered unethical?

The principle would require that a person's medical need establishes his or her moral claim on the attention of persons with medical training. Obviously, this principle is not equivalent to an ethical obligation to respond to every request; it would be physically impossible and financially ruinous for the practitioner. Thus, if it is a principle, it must be limited in some way. The most obvious limits are choosing a specialty, selecting a geographical area, establishing a practice, and setting prices or a payment policy (which should include, if the overall principle is to be respected, some service at no or low fee). Other limits are clearly reprehensible, such as serving only the rich or persons of one race or religion. These limits make a mockery of the overall principle, since being rich or white or Catholic, for example, have nothing to do with medical need.

The most problematic limitation would be one that excludes certain sorts of genuine, treatable medical needs because the physician finds something unacceptable about the need. For example, the disease renders the patient physically repugnant, the disease is associated with behavior the physician considers immoral, or—and this is the case with AIDS—the disease is dangerous to the physician. Clearly, refus-

Dr. Jonsen is a professor of ethics in medicine and chairman of the Department of Medical History and Ethics at the University of Washington School of Medicine.

ing service for the first two reasons could not be justified, but is personal risk a reasonable excuse from service?

Historically, physicians have regularly exposed themselves to serious risk when they treated the victims of infectious diseases. Physicians who fled from the scenes of epidemics have traditionally been criticized (though not always severely). Even when there is a presumption in favor of accepting risk in order to help those in need, the commonly accepted ethical rules for aiding others must be applied: Aid must be feasible, the risk must be reasonable, and there should be no less-risky alternatives.

The "reasonableness" of the risk in caring for AIDS patients is the question. Reasonableness refers to such things as evidence that the activity is actually dangerous, the probability that evil will occur, and the magnitude of the evil for oneself and for others. Each of these elements must be assessed in light of the best available information and the best common sense about the situation at hand.

The best available information reveals that, in general, health workers are at very low risk of contracting HIV infection by the usual run of patient care activities. The predominant studies confirm this, and of the 10 cases of nosocomial HIV infection reported through July 1987, most represent unusually intense exposure. At the same time, the best available information reveals that the magnitude of the evil is great: There is strong chance that infection will proceed to disease and that disease will lead to death. Thus, the moral quandary: Should I undertake an action which I have a presumed duty to perform, if the action has a low probability of resulting in an evil for me (and others; for example, my spouse) of great magnitude? The best answer to that quandary, in my opinion, is yes. The ethical rationale for that answer is that the duty to care for the sick is a strong one, and the avoidance of danger is a weak excuse from performing that duty unless the danger is imminent. Also, the implications of refusing needed care to certain "dangerous" patients are worrisome. Above all, a life ruled by the strategy of avoiding the low probabilities of even great harm would be a paralyzed life.

The answer would shift from a clear yes to a "probably yes" if the probability of harm increases or if the feasibility of helping decreases. Thus, the anticipation of an unavoidable exposure to significant bleeding, together with the real chance of a puncture wound—as might occur when a surgeon is suturing in an obscured and bloody field—would lend some plausibility to a refusal to treat. Similarly, doubt about the benefits of surgery or about its desirability to the patient, such as the proposal to place arterial access for hemodialysis in a terminally ill and demented AIDS patient, would strengthen the ethical justification of a refusal. Also, there may be imminent danger to unconsenting third parties, as when the surgeon may be pregnant. Thus, there are situations in which a physician or surgeon may make a plausible case that he or she will not treat a patient. However, it is obvious that psychological and emotional factors can heighten the sense of danger, magnify perceived risks, or reduce the apparent need or urgency of treatment. Scrupulous honesty and courage are indispensable adjuncts to such ethical evaluation.

A question less dramatic than actual refusal to treat is the proposal to require a pre-operative test for HIV antibody of all surgical patients. Here the relevant question is what decisions might be faced and what procedures initiated on the basis of information gained by that test. Are there specific maneuvers that might be modified if the patient is antibody-positive? For example, would the surgeon staple rather than suture, use a different technique for hemostasis, proceed more slowly and cautiously, pass instruments differently? If there are safer procedures that could be employed in the more dangerous (to the surgeon) situation, what increase in risk to the patient can be tolerated? Clearly, such reasoning can be part of a rational approach to care, and thus pre-operative testing could be justified. At the same time, in the absence of any rational approach, there is a vivid possibility that information about the patient's infective state could lead to unjustified refusal of needed care.

The conclusions, then, are that there is a strong imperative on physicians to respond to the need of the sick, that that imperative does allow certain limitations, but that a refusal to serve based on fear of disease is not easy to justify. It may be justified in certain situations, but only with sound reasons and honest reasoning.

Even when that reasoning points toward a justification, there are still matters that should give pause. Among these is the reputation of the profession. Refusing treatment in specific cases does cast a shadow on medicine's most precious value, its commitment to altruistic service. The words of a physician writing of the desertion of his colleagues during the Great London Plague of 1665 should be recalled:

> "Every man that undertakes to be of a profession or takes upon him any office must take all parts of it, the good and the evill, the pleasure and the pain, the profit and the inconvenience altogether and not pick and chuse, for ministers must preach, captains must fight and physicians attend the sick."
>
> *Dr. Wm Boghurst, LIMOGRAPHIA*
> *Ed. J. F. Payne, London, 1894, p. 61*

Additional Reading

Jonsen, A.R. 1985. Ethics and AIDS. *Bulletin of the American College of Surgeons* 70:15-18.

Jonsen, A.R., Cooke, M., Koenig, B.A. 1986. AIDS and Ethics. *Issues in Science and Technology* 2:56-65.

Perspectives of a Primary Care Physician on Managing Patients with AIDS

by Julia R. Smith, M.D.

50

As an internist, I have provided primary care in the last two years to five patients with acquired immunodeficiency syndrome (AIDS), several persons with AIDS-related complex (ARC), and a number of men and women whose test results are positive for human immunodeficiency virus (HIV). The issue of AIDS has even touched some of my established patients. Some have requested testing to ease fears of "a casual encounter a few years ago;" a neighbor wanted to advise her 16-year-old daughter about kissing.

My involvement with AIDS and related conditions has challenged me more than any other condition I've encountered to engage the science, the art and the politics of medicine.

The science of AIDS: Information available but sketchy

As a rule, physicians are most comfortable when grounded in the science of medicine. The science of AIDS, however, is evolving so rapidly that we are often uncertain about what we have to offer. There is more information than any generalist can keep up with. Although specific information is readily available by phone from publicly funded AIDS projects (see back cover) and from specialist consultants, the following case illustrates that many questions remain unanswered.

CASE 1

Karen is a health professional. Following the normal delivery of her first child, she learned that she had been transfused with HIV-positive blood two years earlier. Her newborn was seropositive, perhaps reflecting maternal antibody, perhaps perinatal infection. In trying to counsel Karen on the risks to her neonate, it would be possible to offer retrovirus cultures of the newborn's blood. (Positive culture would indicate infection of the newborn, but sensitivity of culture in this setting is unknown.) The risk of perinatal transmission is still uncertain, and the prognosis for the perinatally infected infant is not yet well-defined. In counseling Karen on her own risks of AIDS, the prognosis for an otherwise healthy young woman infected by transfusion is not yet clear.

Dr. Smith is an internist in private practice in Seattle and is a clinical assistant professor of medicine at the University of Washington.

AIDS is the province of primary care

Because of the specialized nature of information on AIDS and its complications, one might consider the disease a subspecialty problem. But for several reasons, I believe the management of persons with AIDS and related conditions falls most naturally into the province of primary care medicine. Many of our patients are concerned and request information about AIDS. AIDS must now be considered in the differential diagnosis of many illnesses. AIDS affects multiple organ systems and thus requires input from several subspecialties, rather than falling solely within the province of any single specialty. Primary care providers can best coordinate the advice of consultants, as well as the case management of a great number of psychosocial problems.

We all must be prepared to answer questions about AIDS and to clarify for patients what they learn from the media or hear discussed in casual conversation. Health maintenance screening of all sexually active people should routinely include questioning about risk factors and education about protective sexual practices.

Many of us will see asymptomatic, antibody-positive persons who will benefit from the usual primary-care screening and advice. However, such patients need emotional support in the midst of the uncertainty of their condition as well as continuity with a physician who can evaluate symptoms and problems as they arise.

Appropriately evaluating symptoms in antibody-positive individuals or in patients with ARC is a major clinical challenge to the primary care provider (see "Clinical Manifestations and Approach to Management of HIV Infection and AIDS" on page 27). When does one suspect *Pneumocystis carinii* pneumonia in the patient with cough, cerebral toxoplasmosis in someone with headache, or treatable intestinal infection in someone with loose stools? How exhaustively should one work up fever, fatigue or nausea? HIV-infected persons can experience viral bronchitis or gastroenteritis, migraine or excessive stress. Considerations that dictate a careful search for opportunistic infection are illustrated by the following patient.

CASE 2

Richard is a 33-year-old, married, seropositive bisexual man with a history of fatigue and frequent bouts of axillary hydradenitis.

He developed a fever to 103 degrees and myalgia without respiratory symptoms. Physical examination was unremarkable, and the illness subsided in five days. High fevers returned three weeks later, along with a mild, dry cough. The chest X-ray was clear but the arterial blood pO2 was 70. Gallium scan showed increased uptake in the lungs, and subsequent bronchoalveolar lavage showed *Pneumocystis carinii*. He received sulfamethoxazole-trimethoprim for one week, developed nausea and vomiting, was switched to pentamidine for two more weeks, and is doing well two months later.

The duration and severity of illness are helpful in evaluating common symptoms. The presence of features of more common illnesses—rhinitis, a typical pattern for tension headache or irritable bowel, or isolation of common pathogens—may help to identify a more benign condition. Clinical evidence that suggests deterioration of the patient's immune function—such as onset of oral thrush or prolonged outbreaks of herpes—might raise suspicion about opportunistic infections. Similarly, decline of total lymphocyte count or T4 cell count is associated with increased risk of such infections. In deciding when to pursue more extensive work-up, physicians may want to consider the treatability of a potential AIDS-related disease. Clinicians must deal with the patient's need for reassurance in deciding how to interpret various symptoms. A phone call to a subspecialist about the extent and timing of work-up may be helpful.

Coordinating subspecialty care

When symptoms unique to AIDS develop, a subspecialist often is needed to assist in diagnosis and in planning therapy. However, the continued central involvement of the primary care provider is most important. Serial problems involving multiple organ systems may require several consultants. The generalist plays the pivotal role in coordinating management, producing continuity throughout, and in assessing various subjective considerations in determining a treatment plan. The following cases illustrate issues in coordinating subspecialty care, in withholding invasive diagnostic studies, and in withdrawing therapy.

C A S E 3

Stephen is a married bisexual man with AIDS that had presented as blurred vision due to cytomegalovirus retinitis. After ophthalmologic evaluation, he was placed on an experimental antiviral drug, DHPG, which his wife administered intravenously at home. He developed an unsteady gait and uncontrolled movements of his arm. Cerebrospinal fluid protein was slightly elevated. Computed tomography (CT) scan was unremarkable, but severe nausea and vomiting led to magnetic resonance imaging (MRI) that showed several lesions in the cerebellum suggestive of infection. Despite treatment for presumptive toxoplasmosis, followup MRI showed possible progression of the lesions. Infectious disease and neurology consultants offered brain biopsy as the only way to identify any potentially treatable disease. Stephen and his wife conferred with me before electing to forego biopsy and receive home terminal care. The couple felt that the potential benefits of finding the cause of only his most recent symptoms would not be worth the additional risks, discomfort and added hospital time for brain biopsy.

C A S E 4

John was a 39-year-old gay man who had been treated for *Pneumocystis carinii* pneumonia. He developed persistent diarrhea, and special examinations of the stool revealed only cryptosporidia. Since opiates failed to control the diarrhea, we administered the experimental drug spiramycin, without response. After two months of worsening symptoms, John was rehospitalized for intravenous hyperalimentation and for fluid and electrolyte replacement. Endoscopy and small bowel biopsy by a gastroenterology consultant revealed no curable causes for the diarrhea. Anticipating death, John arranged for a friend to assume legal guardianship. After four months in hospital requiring six to eight liters of fluid replacement a day, John requested that the intravenous support be discontinued. The orders were written, and he was allowed to die.

Since this experience, I have been able to avoid prolonged hospitalization for two other patients with AIDS by arranging 24-hour nursing care at home for one month and for two and one-half months, until death. In both instances, private insurers agreed to fund home care.

To assist the patient and/or family in choosing between aggressive treatment in the hospital vs. home therapy, or between continued efforts to prolong life vs. comfort measures to support the dying process, we must be familiar with the psychosocial and spiritual elements of the situation as well as with the biomedical (see "Psychosocial Aspects of AIDS" on page 42).

The art of caring for persons with AIDS

The personal involvement required in the "art" of caring for someone with AIDS includes the physician's acceptance, emotional support, and willingness to face the issues of death and dying with these patients, and an openness to learning from them. A prerequisite is honest dealing with our own fears and denial, and with the inevitable sense of helplessness that comes when we have no more science to offer.

For many patients with AIDS, the illness provides an occasion for self-examination, reprioritizing of values, and reconciling unfinished business in their lives. Despite the fatal prognosis, a tremendous amount of healing can happen for persons with AIDS and those around them.

If the traditional definition of health refers only to the absence of physical disease, then healing is no longer possible for those with HIV-related conditions. But the healing that occurs for many persons with AIDS is a sense of wholeness (the root word of "health") that results from accepting and integrating all the facets of one's self, even in the face of disability and death.

Technology in this setting takes on a new purpose: to give the patient more time for this type of healing and to minimize suffering. Our task as primary care providers is to facilitate this process by recognizing its importance, providing emotional support (often just listening), and arranging psychosocial assistance when needed.

Practical matters: Coordinating psychosocial support

Coordinating all available psychosocial services is the practical side to the art of caring for persons with AIDS. While we tend to focus on the mechanics of patient care in the hospital or office, patients spend most of their time at home. There, they discover various functional limitations and face the full trauma of their diagnosis.

It is beyond our capacity as private practitioners to handle all psychosocial issues. In Seattle, we are fortunate to have hospital- and community-based services to oversee such matters. Much of this work also is done by many volunteers primarily from the city's gay and lesbian communities. But even so, greater participation and support from the public at large will be essential to meet the needs of the growing population of persons with AIDS in King County (see "The Public Health Response to AIDS" on page 10). Seattle has a great need to develop housing and skilled nursing facilities for AIDS patients and to make home care assistance more available. Physicians' involvement in lobbying for such services could have great impact on the quality of life available to their patients.

In smaller communities, services must be created by modifying or expanding existing systems. Groups such as the American Red Cross, home care services, community college departments of social work, and the religious community may already provide resources that can serve AIDS patients. Support from businesses and the media can have tremendous influence in developing needed community systems and services. Neighbors, friends and volunteers can act as caseworkers to access these services where a formal system is not developed.

Medical professionals need to be much more active at the outset in smaller communities to lobby, inform and guide community and service agencies in providing adequate care.

Community service and the politics of AIDS

Employing the art of medicine may involve us in the politics of medicine as well. In AIDS, such involvement seems unavoidable. As a physician, I personally feel a responsibility to participate in public education about AIDS and to help dissipate public fear and paranoia about the disease. As long as there is ignorance and fear of the modes of HIV transmission, we face the risk of discriminatory and ineffective public policy decisions. We can no longer identify this disease with a few stigmatized social groups. It is important to understand the virus and its potential effect on us all. Our ability to meet the needs of HIV-infected persons and to effectively educate our populace about preventive measures will only be as great as our acceptance of AIDS as a community problem.

As physicians, we are regarded as sources of authoritative information in such matters. We have an opportunity and a responsibility to take the lead in influencing and shaping AIDS public policy, thereby affecting the course of this epidemic in our society.

National Perspectives on the Primary Care Provider's Role in Health Care Delivery for AIDS

by Samuel C. Matheny, M.D., M.P.H., Charles L. Hostetter, M.D., M.P.H., and C. Everett Koop, M.D., Sc.D.

The media and the scientific literature contain numerous reminders of the relentless progression of the acquired immunodeficiency syndrome (AIDS) epidemic and deliver dire projections of the toll this epidemic will take.

Surveillance reports continue to indicate that AIDS still is found predominantly in certain segments of the population—intravenous drug abusers and homosexual/bisexual men. The geographic distribution of these groups results in a clustering of cases of AIDS and of human immunodeficiency virus (HIV) infection in the major metropolitan areas on the East and West coasts. Logically, physicians in these areas have become more familiar with the treatment of HIV-related conditions than their counterparts in lower-prevalence areas.

We are now observing a shift in the demography of the epidemic, with more cases occurring in heretofore low-prevalence areas.

This shift has significant implications for primary care physicians in these areas. All states have now reported AIDS cases, and the numbers indicate that a redistribution to suburban and rural communities will continue. There may be several reasons for this. An increasing number of cases are being reported that have been contracted through heterosexual activity, with the result that anyone who has sexual contact with multiple partners is now at greater risk of infection. Indications for testing have been expanded, and greater numbers of both symptomatic and asymptomatic patients are being evaluated in ambulatory care settings. Also, many AIDS patients are returning to their families of origin in the terminal stages of their illness. The result is that many smaller communities face the agonizing and sometimes divisive issues surrounding the care of AIDS patients, even though the communities may not be perceived as containing "at-risk" populations.

In summary, a much larger and more diverse segment of the population may now be viewed as being at risk for HIV infection. This reinforces the reality that every primary care physician, regardless of locale, must become familiar with the complex array of clinical manifestations of HIV infection and must be informed about the appropriate treatment and management of these conditions.

Prevention

Preventing viral transmission is the only effective measure currently available to control the HIV epidemic. As stated in the Surgeon General's report: "It (AIDS) can be controlled by changes in personal behavior. It is the responsibility of every citizen to be informed about AIDS and to exercise the appropriate preventive measures."

Since physicians generally occupy a unique and trusted position in their patients' eyes, it is the physician's responsibility—both within the individual practice and in the general community—to provide accurate information concerning healthy and unhealthy behaviors. The primary physician may be the most influential and knowledgeable person in the community to work with schools, civic organizations and health groups to disseminate information, to correct misinformation, and to allay fears of contagion.

Testing and clinical management

Much controversy continues to surround the matter of testing for HIV antibody, and many of the issues remain unresolved. Nevertheless, physicians who understand the significance of testing can offer their patients useful information concerning the results, but also must offer counseling. These physicians are in a position to provide an extremely important service. Counseling is an essential part of the serology testing process, whether the patient is seronegative or seropositive, and counseling sessions may be required over an extended period. Seronegative patients must be counseled to stay that way. Seropositive patients must be made aware of their life-saving responsibility to protect others.

The primary care physician also will become more involved with the care of patients who are clinically ill with HIV infection. This will occur of necessity as ever-increasing numbers of patients place demands on the health care system. With more therapeutic options, it is likely that fewer patients will require lengthy hospital stays, and outpatient care will increasingly become the preferred treatment option.

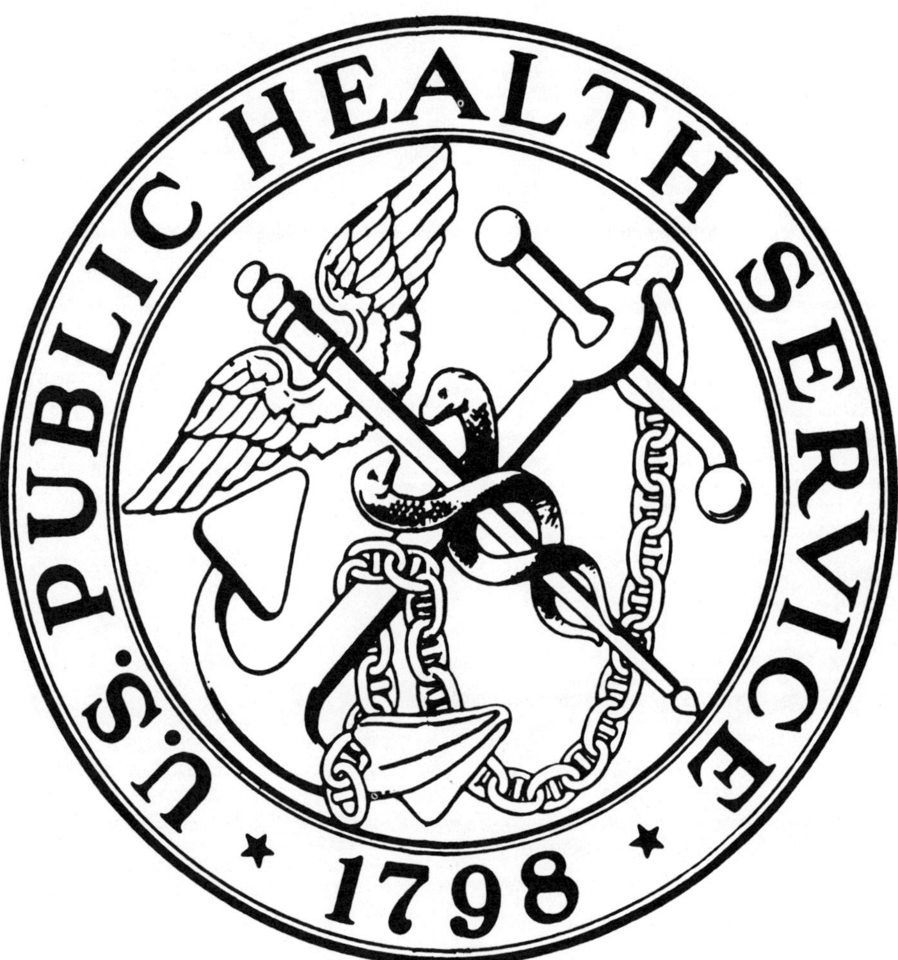

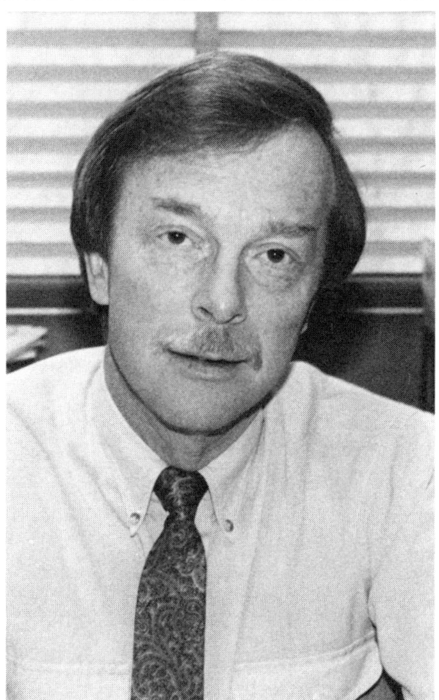

Dr. Matheny is director of the Office of Special Projects in the Health Resources and Services Administration of the U.S. Public Health Service, Rockville, MD.

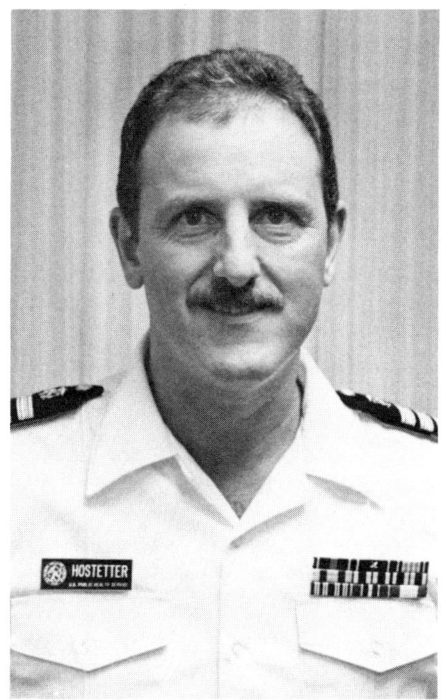

Dr. Hostetter is assistant regional health administrator for state operations in Region IX of the U.S. Public Health Service, San Francisco, CA.

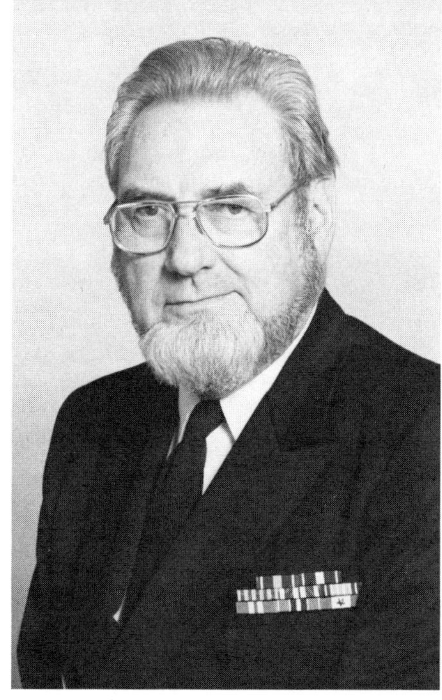

Dr. Koop is the Surgeon General of the U.S. Public Health Service, Washington, D.C.

The involution and debilitation of the AIDS patient are similar in many ways to those processes in the elderly population. They require an approach to care that emphasizes coordination and integration of a spectrum of medical and support services. Institutions with expertise in caring for the elderly and terminally ill are ideal settings for the care of AIDS patients. It is also fortuitous that the recent enhanced interest in geriatrics as part of the medical school curriculum has improved medical residents' skills in the assessment of debilitated patients, recognition of common psychosocial issues, and awareness of the importance of integrating all facets of health care delivery for the fragile patient.

Problems

Although it seems obvious that the primary care physician should have a central role in treating HIV infection, relatively few physicians in each community are caring for the majority of AIDS patients. This situation has been attributed to a number of factors. The disease was originally most prevalent among homosexual men in major urban centers. Even prior to the onset of the epidemic, these men may have specifically sought out health care providers in whom they could confide information concerning their sexuality. On the other hand, many intravenous drug abusers in inner cities lack a primary medical care provider and use the public hospitals and outpatient clinics when illness occurs. With patient numbers increasing and with thousands more "at-risk" patients seeking advice and counseling, the relatively small number of providers currently caring for these patients has already reached the saturation point in some areas.

Needs

For AIDS care to enter the mainstream of primary medical care, physicians must be able to recognize patients who are at risk or who practice high-risk behaviors, to counsel appropriately, and to make realistic recommendations for behavior modification. Information concerning the appropriateness of specific laboratory tests, the correct interpretation of these tests, and the initiation of indicated therapy must be understood and made part of the physician's clinical armamentarium. Physicians must recognize and internalize the fact that AIDS, even though it is presently incurable, is not untreatable.

It is equally important that new developments in diagnosis and therapy be disseminated in a manner that will reassure primary care physicians of their ability to stay abreast of new information. When assistance is needed or referrals are indicated, systems for transmitting information among consultants and primary care providers should be streamlined.

Improvements in case management could enormously benefit the primary care physician. As in the case of geriatric patients, the patient with AIDS may have critical needs for prompt use of a variety of services requiring the coordination of a diverse number of providers, from home care to legal services. If the needs of primary physicians are considered when these case management systems are designed, the quality of services that a physician can render may significantly improve.

The federal response

The U.S. Public Health Service has recognized the unique concerns of those who provide primary care services for people with AIDS and other HIV-related conditions, and has developed plans to prepare primary care professionals to meet this challenge. A strategy has been developed that provides for regular and frequent liaison among representatives of the five U.S. Public Health Service agencies to coordinate AIDS activities and identify deficiencies, including training of health professionals.

The Health Resources and Services Administration, for example, has funded the first four of 10 education and training centers to work with a range of health professionals, providing educational programs and on-site clinical experience in a variety of settings. The UW received one of these grants for $1.7 million to establish such a center, which will provide AIDS training for an estimated 7,500 health care professionals affiliated with larger clinics and hospitals in Washington, Alaska, Montana, Idaho and Oregon. Programs at the centers will be tailored to the needs of the specific communities and the educational priorities of the participants. These centers also are intended to serve as clearinghouses for educational materials that practitioners can use in caring for individual patients and in community education.

In a similar manner, the National Institute of Mental Health has developed a number of Education and Training Centers to provide specific information and training in various areas of interest to physicians, such as counseling, diagnosis and treatment of mental health problems that accompany HIV infection. The National Institute of Drug Abuse develops and sponsors training activities aimed specifically at health care professionals involved in drug abuse therapy programs. Prevention of HIV transmission among intravenous drug abusers is a major emphasis of these programs.

The Centers for Disease Control, through 10 Sexually Transmitted Disease Prevention/Training Centers, provides training in HIV epidemiology, prevention and control for a range of health care professionals. Estimates are that 600 to 800 professionals will be trained this year in these centers, one of which is based at the University of Washington School of Medicine.

The National Institutes of Health also provides training to health care professionals, emphasizing research updates in the fields of virology, immunology, vaccine development and therapeutics. For example, 500 participants from the Northwest attended a seminar, "AIDS: Practical Application for Nurses and Social Workers," that the National Institute of Allergy and Infectious Diseases sponsored at the UW in August.

Equally important is the cooperative spirit that a number of professional organizations—such as the American Medical Association and the American Osteopathic Association—have exhibited in responding to the need for professional support and education. The U.S. Public Health Service has co-sponsored meetings and seminars and has worked with task forces in these organizations to prepare physicians for the complex issues that lie ahead.

The HIV epidemic is a national problem. Its impact goes beyond jurisdictional, ethnic, racial or gender barriers. The national response must enlist our untiring individual and collective efforts. Partnerships of federal, state, county and municipal government entities; the private health care sector; health professions organizations representing all disciplines, and health professions training institutions are essential if we are to successfully meet this challenge. As in past public health crises, primary care physicians play a central role in this epidemic by providing leadership, both in prevention of transmission and in the compassionate care of those who are ill.

The opinions published herein are those of the authors and not necessarily those of the federal government.

Additional Reading

U.S. Department of Health and Human Services, Public Health Service, Health Resources and Services Administration. 1987. *Surgeon General's Report on Acquired Immune Deficiency Syndrome.*

Infection Control in AIDS

by Patricia Lynch, R.N., and Walter E. Stamm, M.D.

Since the onset of the acquired immunodeficiency syndrome (AIDS) epidemic, nosocomial transmission of the human immunodeficiency virus (HIV) to health care workers has been a major concern. As of July 1987, nine hospital-based health care workers and one dentist in the United States reportedly had acquired HIV infection in the course of their work. None has developed AIDS. Nosocomial transmission of HIV to other patients or visitors has been neither reported nor suspected in any health care setting. These data clearly indicate that the risk of nosocomial HIV transmission is very low. Nonetheless, health care workers are understandably concerned (and sometimes fearful) about their personal risk and are universally eager to employ whatever infection prevention strategies might be effective for themselves, patients and visitors. Some of the major questions regarding nosocomial infections and AIDS include:

—Are health care workers likely to become infected by caring for patients with AIDS, and if so, how?

—Are health care workers likely to become infected with the opportunistic infections characteristic of AIDS patients?

—Are patients likely to become infected when cared for by a health care worker with HIV infection?

—What circumstances might lead to indirect transmission of HIV through use of shared equipment?

—Are other patients (particularly roommates) or visitors at risk for nosocomial transmission of HIV or opportunistic infections?

Although direct answers to these questions are not yet available, the risks of HIV transmission in the hospital and possible prevention strategies are becoming increasingly clear. We review them here.

The parallel with hepatitis B virus infection

In the early 1980s, several studies confirmed what anecdotes had long suggested: that health care workers in some occupational categories were much more likely to have serologic evidence of hepatitis B virus infection than a randomly selected population, such as volunteer blood donors. Occupational exposure to blood was identified as the major risk factor associated with hepatitis B virus acquisition in health

Ms. Lynch is an infection control practitioner at Harborview Medical Center and an adjunct clinical instructor of epidemiology at the University of Washington. Dr. Stamm is head of Harborview's Infectious Diseases Division and is a UW professor of medicine and an adjunct professor of epidemiology.

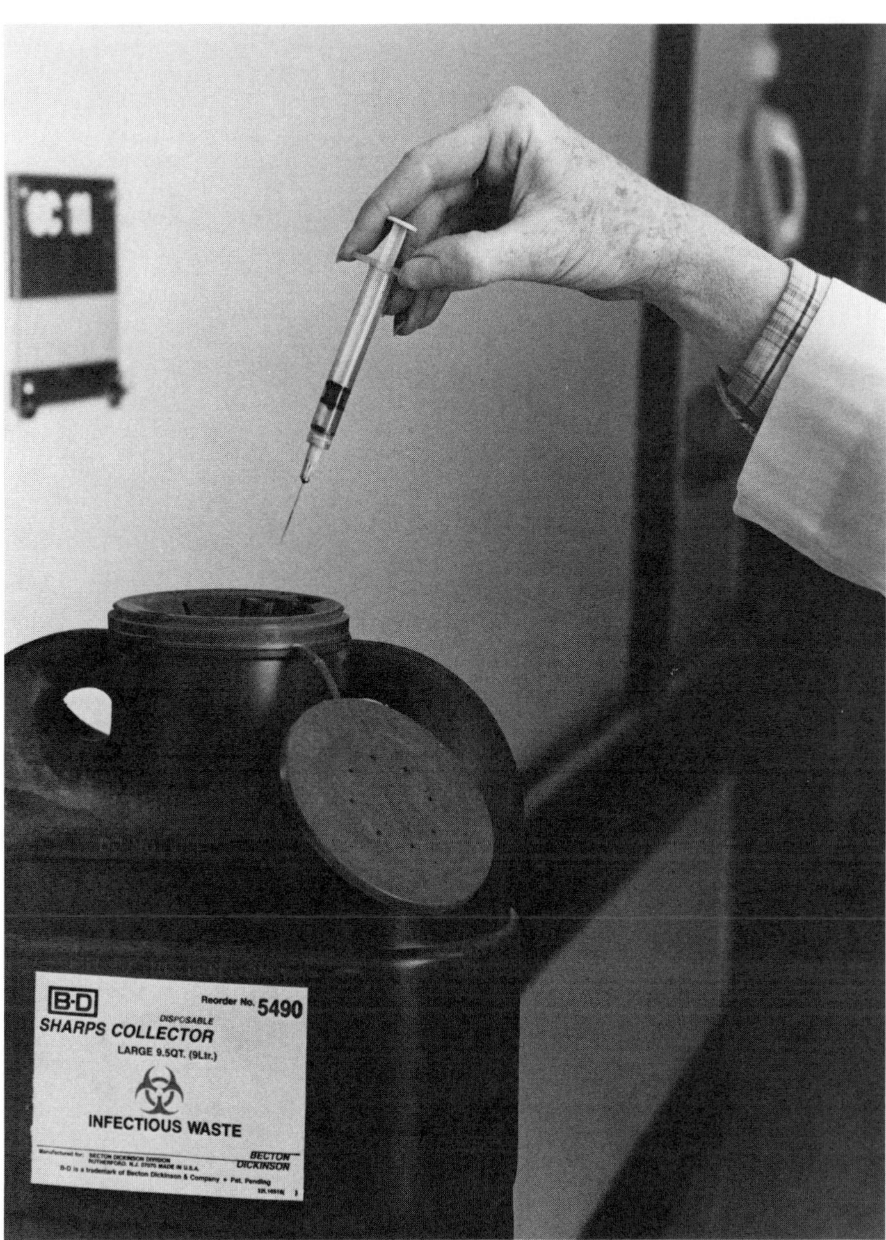

FIGURE 1. To avoid the risk of needlestick transmission of HIV, used needles should not be capped or manipulated before disposal in a puncture-resistant container.

care workers. Thus, highest rates of hepatitis B virus infection were observed in emergency ward nurses, pathologists, dentists, laboratory staff and surgeons. Lower rates were observed in ward nurses and medical house staff. Patients also acquired hepatitis B virus from infected health care workers under some circumstances, usually during invasive procedures such as surgery or dentistry. Occasionally, inadequately disinfected equipment—for example, endoscopes or dialysis ma-

chines—appeared to play a role in hepatitis B virus transmission.

Like hepatitis B virus, HIV is present in blood and other body secretions such as semen and, in lesser quantities, saliva and urine. Both viruses also are transmitted though sexual and blood contact. Thus, it is easy to understand why health care workers are concerned about nosocomial HIV acquisition. If HIV and hepatitis B virus are transmitted by the same routes, and if the same infection-prevention strategies that have been relatively unsuccessful for

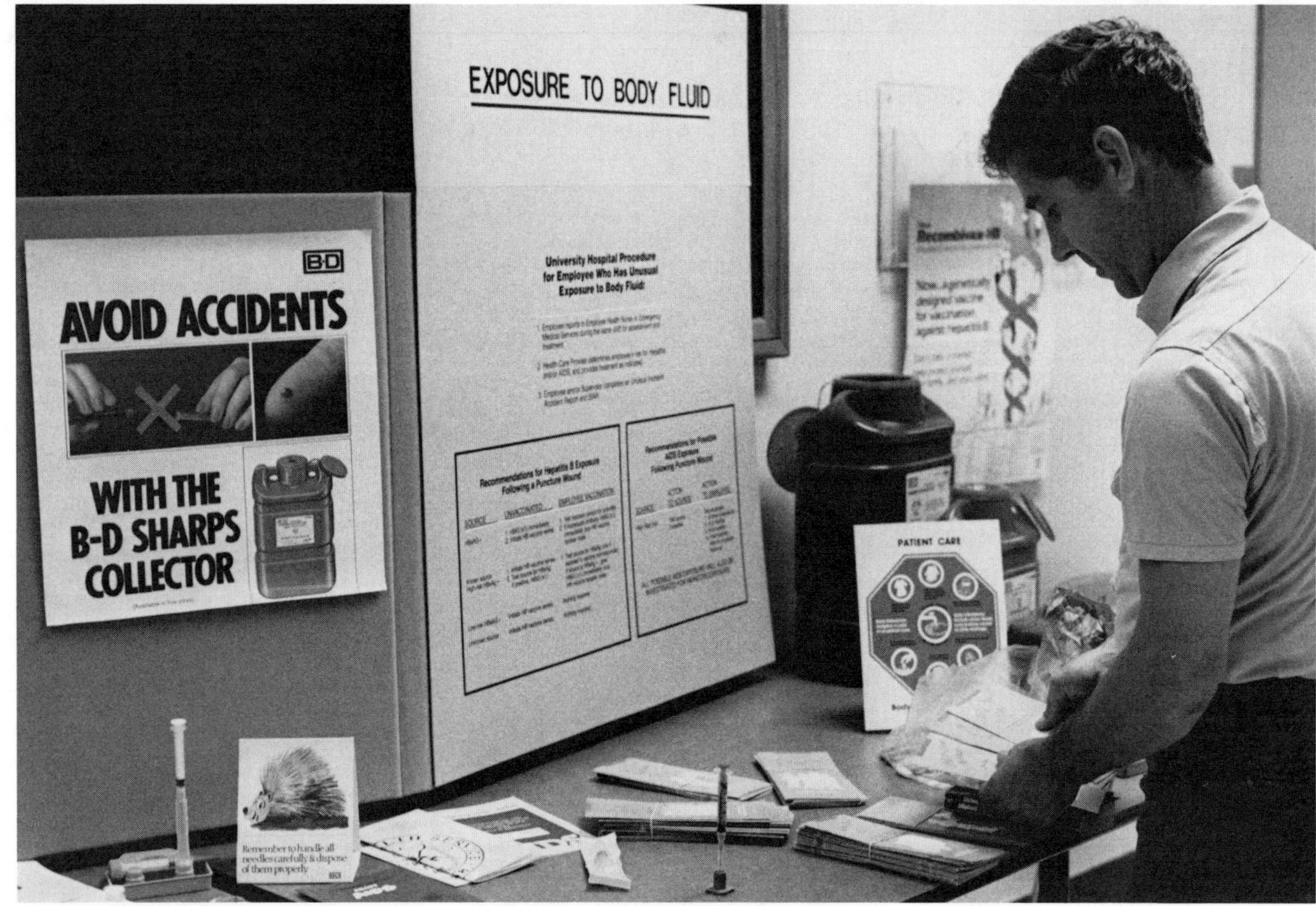

FIGURE 2. University of Washington Hospital employees learn about the appropriate use and disposal of sharp medical instruments during "Sharps Awareness Week."

hepatitis B virus are used for HIV, then the risk of HIV transmission would seem substantial.

These two diseases share the same routes of transmission but, fortunately, are not spread with equal ease. After a needlestick exposure to an infected patient's blood, the risk of hepatitis B virus transmission is 25 to 30 percent, while the risk of HIV transmission is less than 1 percent (Figure 1). A partial explanation for this difference may be that the blood of HIV-infected persons appears to have far fewer infectious particles than the blood of a person infected with hepatitis B virus, reducing the likelihood of transmission from an average inoculum. Other viral and host factors may also be important.

Risk of HIV transmission from an infected patient to health care workers

Several studies have reported results of monitoring more than 1,700 hospital personnel for HIV acquisition after needlestick injuries or mucous membrane exposures to known AIDS patients; three employees without other risk factors may have seroconverted. To date, there have been reports of nine health care workers in whom nosocomial HIV infection is believed to have occurred, and all had occupational exposure to blood. In two workers, the blood exposure was unusually prolonged or extensive. Four of the health care workers were punctured with contaminated needles; two of these persons were inadvertently injected with small volumes of the patients' blood. In one case, spattered blood was ingested and in two cases, broken skin may have played a role in acquisition. Several of the patients involved were not known to have AIDS when the health care worker exposure occurred.

Since the epidemic began, approximately 45,000 people have met the definition of AIDS. Most of those patients have been hospitalized at least once, generating hundreds of thousands of patient-caregiver contacts. Except for the nine cases mentioned previously, no transmission to personnel, visitors or other patients has been documented. No cases of HIV infection have been suspected or proven to be related to non-sexual or non-parenteral contact, including bites from infected patients. In a large study of household contacts of AIDS patients, no HIV infection was transmitted even though some household members shared the patients' razors and toothbrushes (see "Epidemiology of AIDS and HIV Infection in the United States and the Pacific Northwest" on page 5).

Transmission of opportunistic infections

AIDS patients develop frequent and recurrent opportunistic infections (see "Clinical Manifestations and Approach to Management of HIV Infection and AIDS" on page 27). The severity of their illnesses makes hospital personnel question whether the infectious agents are particularly virulent or readily transmissible. In fact, most infections in AIDS patients are opportunistic pathogens that infect only individuals with inadequate immune function. Thus, the risk to healthy hospital employees of infection with *Pneumocystis carinii*, *Mycobacterium avium-intracellulare*, toxoplasmosis, or cryptococcosis is negligible. Other pathogens that commonly cause opportunistic infections in AIDS patients—including herpes simplex virus, varicella-zoster virus, candida and cytomegalovirus—already have infected many "normal" individuals. In AIDS patients, such infections recrudesce and disseminate; in persons with a healthy immune system, they remain dormant.

Although no cases of patients, visitors or health care workers acquiring opportunistic infections from AIDS patients have been reported, three infections commonly seen in AIDS patients could cause nosocomial infections in health care workers. AIDS patients are at increased risk for tuberculosis, and hospitals that care for AIDS patients should routinely give personnel tuberculin tests. Hospitals also should place patients with tuberculosis in private rooms, and use improved ventilation systems and ultraviolet ceiling lights to reduce the transmission risk. Transmission of herpes simplex virus or varicella-zoster from extensive mucocutaneous lesions to health care workers' unprotected fingers can produce herpetic whitlow. All health care workers dealing with such skin lesions should wear gloves.

Precautions to prevent transmission of HIV and opportunistic infections:

What precautions are reasonable and for whom should they be used?

Several recent news stories have highlighted the issue of precautions to prevent HIV transmission. In Washington, D.C., police assisting with traffic and crowd control wore rubber gloves when working near the hotel where the Third International AIDS Conference was held in June. In New York, jurors and court attendants wore masks and rubber gloves while a man with AIDS was on trial. Garbage collectors in Boston refuse to pick up trash from the local AIDS Project office. In a fairly large survey of house staff, respondents thought they were at risk for acquiring AIDS and should be allowed to refuse to care for AIDS patients. Appropriate infection precautions must be aimed at preventing known avenues of transmission, but educating personnel to eliminate unfounded fears is also of great importance (Figure 2).

Traditionally, hospitals have focused on using precautions for known cases of disease. This approach presumes that most infective cases can be readily recognized and diagnosed. Unfortunately, this is not true of AIDS nor of many other infectious diseases. For this reason, the concept of identifying known cases and then taking extra precautions with just those cases may actually lead to a false sense of security and to relaxation of precautions with other patients, and thus may facilitate transmission from unrecognized cases.

Screening for HIV as a basis for precautions

The San Francisco AIDS Task Force discussed the value of screening all hospital patients for HIV and concluded that it is preferable to use infection precautions for contact with blood and body substances from all patients. This approach improves the overall standard of care and insures that precautions are not relaxed for patients with negative test results who might later be infectious. The Centers for Disease Control also suggests that this strategy be followed in dental offices and when performing invasive procedures. Additional disadvantages of screening include expense, low yield, and occasional false-negative and false-positive results.

A generic approach to infection control: Body substance isolation

Since HIV infections often go clinically unrecognized, precautions taken just with blood and body substances of individuals known to be infected will not adequately protect personnel. Instead, precautions must be taken with all patients.

At Harborview Medical Center in Seattle, this strategy has been used exclusively since 1985. The key elements of the system, called body substance isolation, are:

—Wear gloves when contact with any patient's mucous membranes, non-intact skin or moist body substances is likely.

—Wash hands before patient contact and whenever (despite gloving) soiling occurs.

—Wear gowns or plastic aprons when it is likely that health care worker clothing will be soiled by moist body substances from any patient.

—Wear masks, goggles, glasses, hair covers or other barriers as necessary to protect personnel from splashing or soiling.

—Use private rooms for patients who extensively soil the room with moist body substances or who have airborne communicable diseases. AIDS patients do not routinely need private rooms.

—Place all used "sharps"—needles or other instruments capable of cutting or puncturing—in rigid containers and autoclave them before disposal.

—Handle trash and soiled linen from all patients uniformly: Put heavily soiled linen through a cold-water rinse cycle before washing. Bag trash securely and dispose in keeping with facility policy and regulatory agency requirements.

—Handle all laboratory specimens as if the patient were known to be infective.

Every patient room has a sign outlining these precautions (Figure 3). For patients with communicable diseases that can be transmitted by air, an additional room sign requests check-in at the nurses' station before entering so that susceptible people can be kept out. To help keep the patient's diagnosis confidential, signs do not identify the patient's disease and precautions do not depend on diagnosis (except with airborne communicable diseases).

This system of precautions offers substantial protection to personnel but is a major change from the diagnosis-dependent isolation systems that many hospitals have used for years. Personnel need to glove

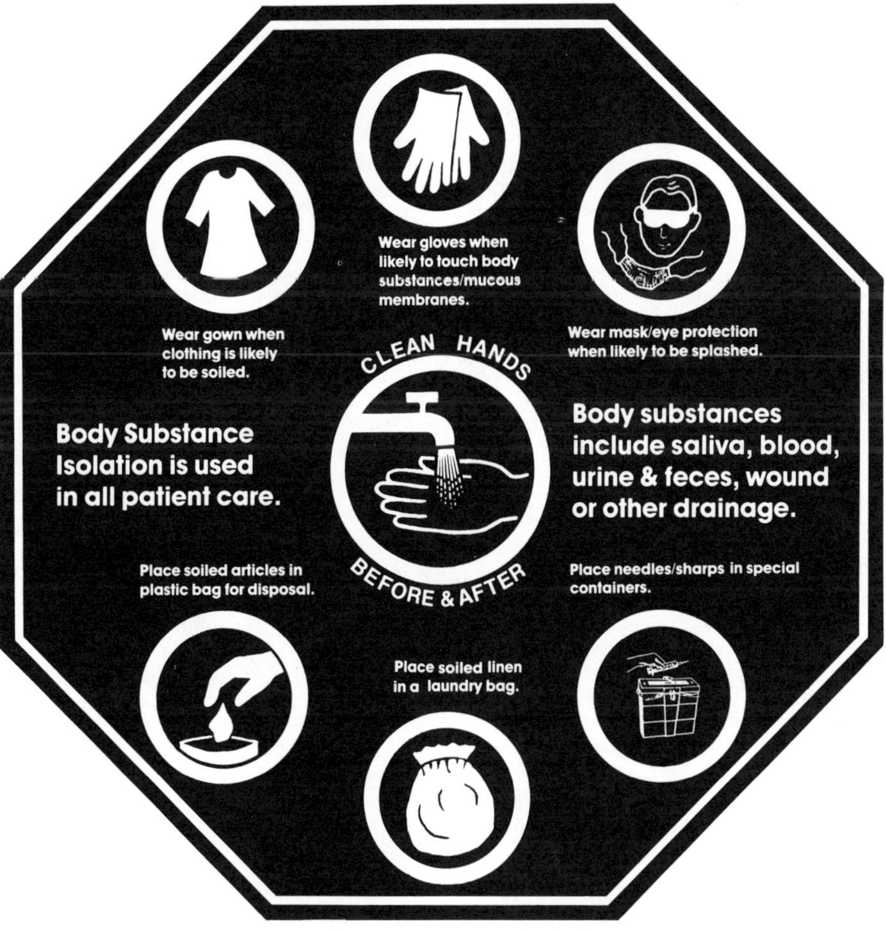

FIGURE 3. This poster, developed at Seattle's Harborview Medical Center, reminds hospital staff about body substance isolation procedures for all patients.

more frequently, creating a challenge to inspire physicians and other health care workers to comply. In general, our medical staff has accepted this system as easy to understand because the rationale is clear, and easy to implement because it eliminates many of the categories and category-specific practices of previous systems.

Ineffective practices

Gowns, masks, gloves or other protective barriers are not needed unless contact with a patient's mucous membranes, non-intact skin or moist body substances is likely. Excessive use should be discouraged. The use of disposable plates and eating utensils is not beneficial and gives patients cold, unattractive meals. Protective isolation—as practiced in general hospitals—neither prolongs life nor decreases the number of infections in compromised hosts.

Precautions for special circumstances

Invasive procedures include all surgical, dental, obstetric and other procedures that involve entry into tissues, cavities or organs. No cases of HIV transmission from a patient to a health care worker—except for the reported case of the dentist—or from a health care worker to a patient during an invasive procedure have been reported. The following precautions are recommended by the Centers for Disease Control:

—Health care workers must wear gloves when touching mucous membranes or non-intact skin of all patients and use other barriers when indicated (for example, masks and goggles if body fluids are likely to be aerosolized). Gloves should be changed between patients and when glove punctures or tears occur.

—After use, disposable syringes and needles, scalpels and other sharps must be placed in puncture-resistant containers. Needles should not be recapped or manipulated.

—No health care worker with exudative lesions or weeping dermatitis should perform or assist in invasive procedures or other direct patient-care activity or handle equipment used for patient care.

Exposure management

Health care workers with parenteral or mucous membrane exposure to patients' blood should report the incident to the appropriate hospital department. Similarly, if a patient has parenteral or mucous membrane exposure to a health care worker's blood, the patient should be told of the incident. Subsequent management recommendations are the same for both groups:

—The donor source should be identified and informed. The recipients should be evaluated and treated prophylactically for hepatitis B if indicated.

—The donor may be screened for HIV after giving consent.

—The recipient should be counseled and screened for HIV as soon as possible after the incident to establish baseline information. Recipients found to be HIV positive need not be screened again. Recipients who are serologically negative should be screened again at three-, six- and 12-month intervals after the incident. Seroconversion is believed to occur usually within three months.

Laboratory practices

Laboratories should adhere to P2-level containment procedures for all specimens. This involves wearing gloves when the hands are likely to be soiled with any specimen, wearing lab coats or disposable gowns when clothing is likely to be soiled, and using other barriers such as masks and goggles when aerosolization is likely (Figure 4). Mouth pipetting, smoking and eating at the benches is prohibited. Blood spills are cleaned by gloved personnel using a disinfectant approved as tuberculocidal.

Many hospitals use biohazard labels for blood or other specimens being sent to the laboratory from patients with AIDS, hepa-

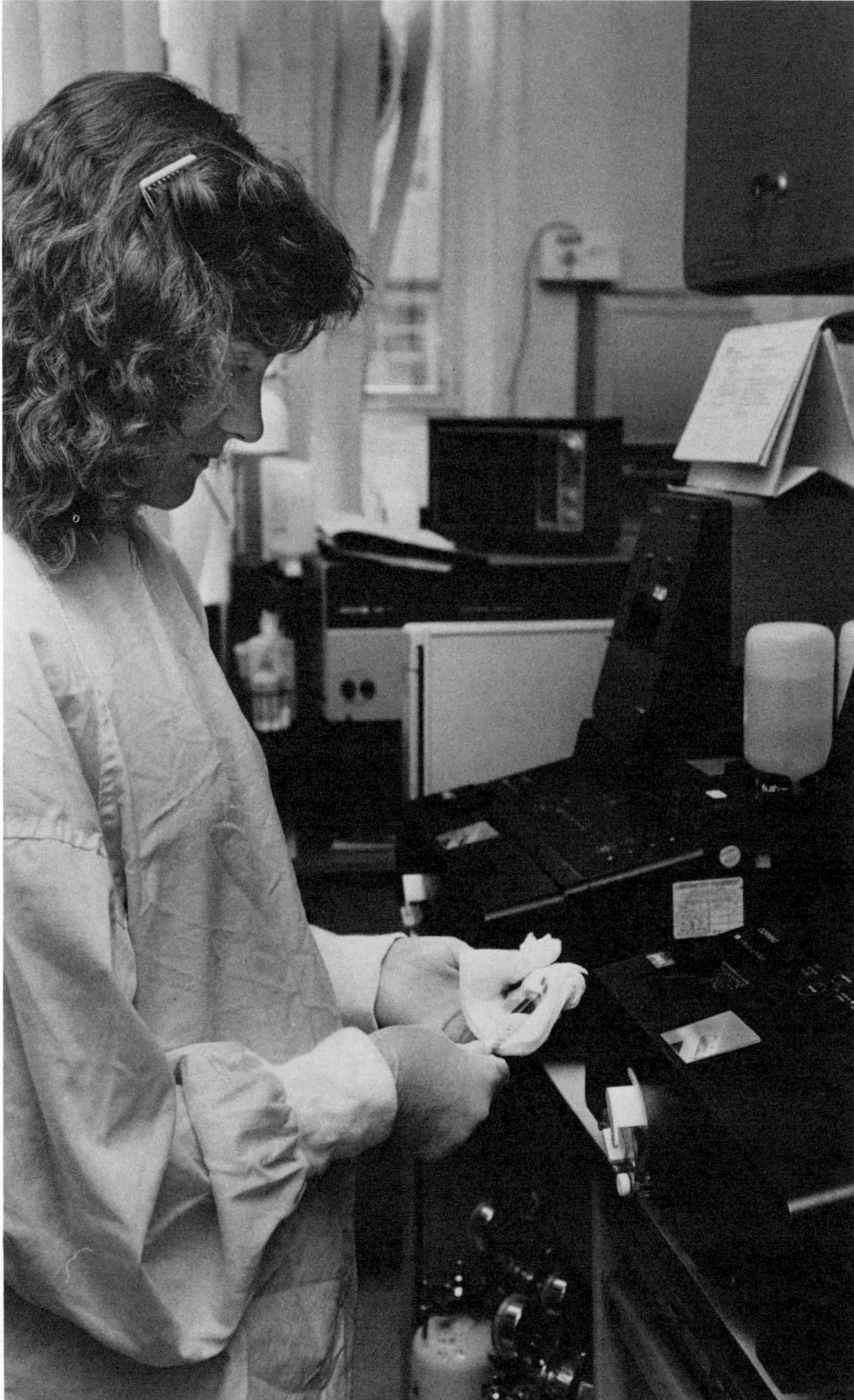

FIGURE 4. Debra Mantyla, a medical technologist in the chemistry laboratory at Harborview Medical Center in Seattle, is gloved and gowned in accordance with P2-level containment procedures.

titis B virus or other infections. This policy has the same shortcomings as disease-specific isolation precautions: Because many infections are not clinically apparent, labels are not affixed to all potentially infectious specimens. The high rate of hepatitis B transmission in laboratory workers may reflect in part the failure of such labeling practices. In our view, all specimens entering the laboratory must be considered potentially infectious and handled with appropriate precautions.

Resuscitation

Mechanical resuscitation equipment (Ambu bags) should be readily available in all health care facilities. No cases of seroconversion following oral resuscitation of an HIV-infected patient have been reported, but use of mechanical equipment is preferable.

Health care workers with HIV infection

Health care workers infected with hepatitis B occasionally have transmitted the infection to patients, usually while performing invasive procedures. This phenomenon has not yet been reported with AIDS and probably is less likely to occur, but it seems prudent that health care workers with HIV infection avoid participating in invasive procedures. Routine patient care probably can be safely provided by HIV-seropositive health care workers who are otherwise healthy and do not have open lesions.

Summary

Current data suggest that a health care worker's risk of HIV infection from an infected patient is small but certainly present. Needlestick injuries or other direct exposures to blood from HIV-positive patients account for the cases reported to date, and preventive measures to reduce the occurrence of these specific events are of great importance. Casual contact does not result in HIV transmission from patients to health care workers, and most opportunistic infections of AIDS patients pose little risk to health care workers. Health care workers should use appropriate precautions for anticipated contacts with the blood or secretions of any hospitalized patient, not just those having AIDS or any other infection.

Additional Reading

Centers for Disease Control. 1987. Update: Human immunodeficiency virus infections in health-care workers exposed to blood of infected patients. *Morbid Mortal Weekly Rep* 36:285-289.

Centers for Disease Control. 1985. Update: Evaluation of human lymphotropic virus type III/lymphadenopathy-associated virus infection in health-care personnel-United States. *Morbid Mortal Weekly Rep* 34:575-578.

Centers for Disease Control. 1987. Recommendations for prevention of HIV transmission in health-care settings. *Morbid Mortal Weekly Rep Supplement 2* 36:1S-19S.

Centers for Disease Control. 1986. Recommended infection control practices for dentistry. *Morbid Mortal Weekly Rep* 35:237-242.

Dienstag, J.L., Ryan, K.M. 1982. Occupational exposure to hepatitis B virus in hospital personnel: Infection or immunization. *Am J Epidemiol* 115:26-39.

Gerberding, J.L. *et al.* 1986. Recommended infection control policies for patients with human immunodeficiency virus infection: An update. *N Engl J Med* 315:1562-1564.

Lynch, P., Jackson, M.M., Cummings, M.J., Stamm, W.E. Rethinking the role of isolation practices in preventing nosocomial infections. *Ann Intern Med*, in press.

A Global Perspective on AIDS

by Joan Kreiss, M.D., M.S.P.H., and King K. Holmes, M.D., Ph.D.

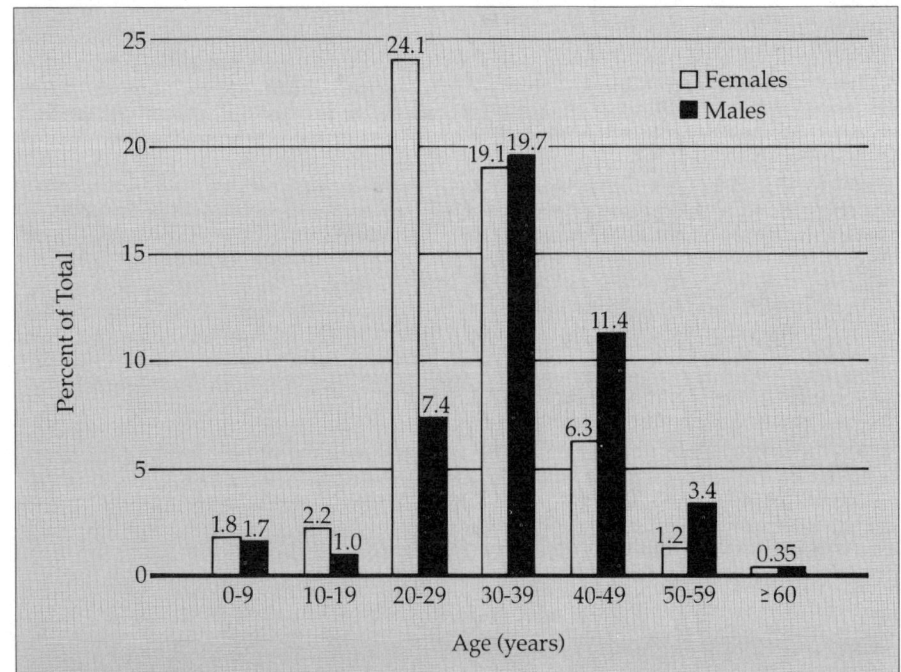

FIGURE 1. The distribution by age and sex of the first 500 AIDS cases diagnosed in Kinshasa, Zaire, between August 1985 and December 1985. Female cases were significantly younger than male cases. Women accounted for the majority of AIDS cases in the age group 20-29, whereas men accounted for the majority of cases in the age groups 40-49 and 50-59.

By early 1987, an estimated 100,000 cases of acquired immunodeficiency syndrome (AIDS) had occurred worldwide, with perhaps 5 million to 10 million people infected by human immunodeficiency viruses. Two distinct human immunodeficiency viruses have been discerned in Africa. HIV-1 (the type implicated in all cases of AIDS in the United States so far) is epidemic in Central Africa and East Africa. HIV-2 has recently been discovered to be widespread in West Africa. Antibodies to HIV-1 were first detected in a blood specimen collected in Central Africa in 1959 (see related article). The first recognized cases of AIDS occurred in the mid-1970s in Central Africa, where HIV-1 has spread quickly, mainly by heterosexual contact. Ten to 20 percent of the young adult population of some cities in Zaire, Rwanda, Uganda, Zambia, the Congo and Tanzania have been infected, and many if not most of those infected will die of AIDS. The prevalence rates of HIV infection have been much lower in the rural areas of these countries, particularly those that are remote from interurban highways.

Spread of HIV-1 in Africa has been fostered by rapid population growth, rural-urban migration, disintegration of traditional cul-

tures, and other factors contributing to prostitution and heterosexual promiscuity. Genital ulcer disease, especially chancroid, promotes sexual transmission of HIV in Africa. In West Africa, HIV-2 has been found in highest prevalence in prostitutes, and therefore is also probably spread by heterosexual transmission. It is now accepted that HIV-2, like HIV-1, causes AIDS. In industrial countries such as the United States, HIV-1 is spread primarily by homosexual contact and intravenous drug abuse. In Latin America, where Brazil and Mexico have reported the largest number of cases of AIDS, patterns of transmission of HIV so far resemble those seen in the United States. In Asia, patterns of spread are not yet defined. Assuming no vaccine, drug therapy, or major behavioral change within four years, there will by conserva-

tive estimate be 50 million to 100 million people worldwide with HIV infection by 1991.

Epidemiology of AIDS in Africa

Heterosexual transmission: Possible lessons

Heterosexual transmission accounts for the vast majority of HIV infection in adults in Africa, but still accounts for a relatively small proportion (4 percent) of U.S. cases. Thus, the ratio of males to females with AIDS is approximately 1:1 in Africa vs. greater than 10:1 in industrialized countries. In the initial study of HIV infection in Rwanda, 69 percent of cases occurred in prostitutes or heterosexually promiscuous men or their wives. In subsequent studies, prostitutes have been identified as high-risk persons, both in Africa and in the developed world. The prevalences of serum antibody to HIV in prostitute communities have ranged from 88 percent in Butare, Rwanda; to 66 percent in Nairobi, Kenya; 37 percent in Bukoba, Tanzania; and 27 percent in Kinshasa, Zaire. In the United States, the prevalence of antibody is also high in some groups of prostitutes, but this appears to be more attributable to intravenous drug abuse than to sexual transmission. In Africa, illicit use of intravenous drugs has not contributed to the epidemic.

Studies of African men attending sexually transmitted disease (STD) clinics—many of whom have had sexual contact with prostitutes—demonstrate that prostitutes are important reservoirs and disseminators of infection. Antibody to HIV was found in 8 percent of such men in Nairobi, Kenya; 28 percent in Butare, Rwanda; and 29 percent in Lusaka, Zambia. In a prospective study at a Nairobi STD clinic of men with genitourinary complaints following recent prostitute contact, 16 (8 percent) of 199 initially seronegative men developed antibody to HIV over the following two to six months. This extraordinary rate of female-to-male transmission is much higher than previously estimated from most U.S. studies.

Dr. Kreiss is assistant professor of medicine and of epidemiology at the University of Washington. Dr. Holmes is chief of Harborview Medical Center's Department of Medicine and is professor and vice-chairman of the UW Department of Medicine.

Table I Prevalence of HIV Antibody in Blood Donors, Hospital Workers and Pregnant Women in Selected African Cities

	Blood donors	Hospital workers	Pregnant women
Kampala, Uganda	11%	NA	14%
Lusaka, Zambia	18%	19%	9%
Kigali, Rwanda	18%	18%	NA
Kinshasa, Zaire	6%	6%	8%
Nairobi, Kenya	NA	2%	3%

Why is heterosexual transmission so much more important in Africa than in developed countries? Answers may include differences in heterosexual behavior, including a much greater frequency of prostitution in Africa, and the existence of cofactors that facilitate sexual transmission in Africa. Four studies in Kenya have found that genital ulcer disease is correlated with increased risk of HIV infection. In the most conclusive of these studies, a cohort of seronegative prostitutes was followed prospectively in Nairobi; 64 percent seroconverted within two years, and the odds of seroconversion were three times higher among those experiencing genital ulcers (usually chancroid) during follow-up than among those who remained free of genital ulcers. Since chancroid and syphilis are epidemic throughout many African countries, this may help to explain the epidemic of heterosexually transmitted HIV in Africa. Antibody to herpes simplex virus type 2 and to syphilis has been associated with the presence of antibody to HIV-1 in homosexual men in the United States in two studies at the University of Washington (Corey L., Handsfield H. *et al*, unpublished data), suggesting that rectal and genital ulcers could be cofactors for homosexual transmission of HIV as well.

A recent idea is that HIV carriers may become more infectious over time. Since the AIDS epidemic may be of longer duration in Central Africa than in developed countries, heterosexual transmission may be more efficient in Africa. In early U.S. studies of stable couples in which one member has acquired HIV infection through clotting factor concentrate or blood transfusions, the rate of either female-to-male or male-to-female transmission has been only 10 to 20 percent, even after years of sexual exposure. A recent study suggests that the risk of heterosexual transmission from a hemophiliac to his spouse becomes greater as his peripheral blood T4 lymphocyte count drops. This might be due to an increase in the amount of circulating free virus as the infection progresses. If this is borne out, then differences in observed rates of heterosexual transmission could be related to the stage of HIV infection in the index case. It could be that the efficiency of heterosexual transmission early in the course of the epidemic will be lower than later in the epidemic, when growing numbers of heterosexually active persons will have more advanced HIV infection and immunosuppression.

In Miami, a prospective study of serologically "discordant" couples (one member infected and one uninfected at the beginning of the study) showed seroconversion in 86 percent of those who were repeatedly exposed without use of condoms over a period of two years or less. This ominously high rate of heterosexual transmission resembles that seen in Africa, but has not yet been seen in other U.S. populations.

Other cofactors that facilitate sexual transmission of HIV are less firmly established. In the study of African prostitutes men-

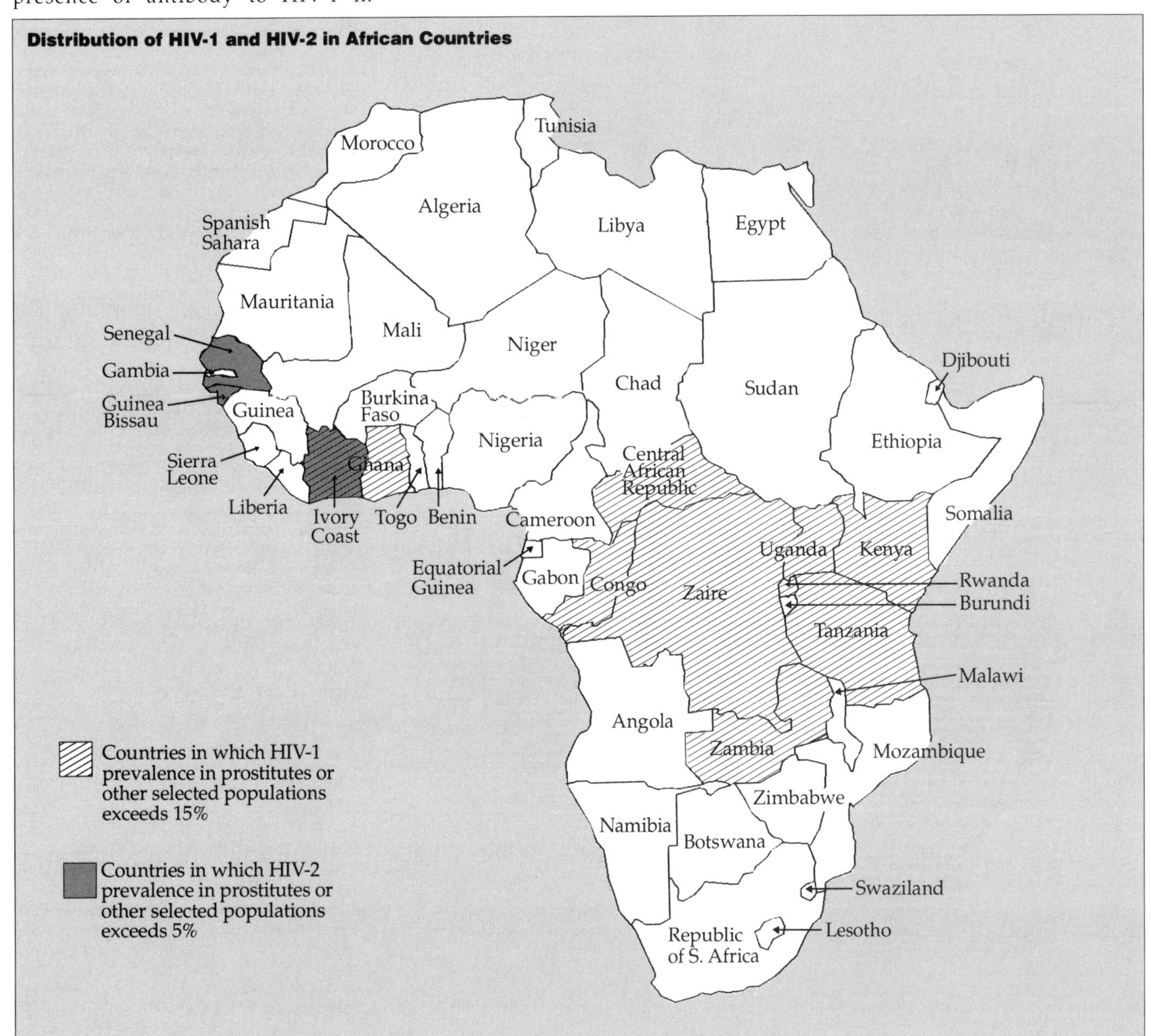

FIGURE 2. The distribution of HIV-1 and HIV-2 in African countries.

tioned above, oral contraceptive use was associated with an increased risk of HIV infection after controlling for covariables. This observation will require corroboration in other populations. Recent studies in homosexual men suggest that genetic factors such as HLA type or group specific component (Gc) phenotype may influence susceptibility to HIV infection or disease progression. Subsequent studies have failed to confirm this. Studies of genetic risk factors for HIV are only beginning in Africa and elsewhere.

Blood transfusion transmission

Blood transfusions are the second major mode of transmission of HIV in Africa. As shown in Table I, seroprevalence rates in blood donors in certain African cities are extremely high: 18 percent in Kigali, Rwanda; 6 percent in Kinshasa, Zaire; and 18 percent in Lusaka, Zambia. For comparison, the prevalence of HIV antibody in U.S. blood donors is 0.1 to .01 percent. From the "look-back" program in this country, which traces recipients of infected blood products administered before HIV screening was available, it appears that receipt of a contaminated unit of blood is associated with a 90-percent risk of infection. Thus, blood transfusion is the most efficient means of HIV transmission.

Anemia is common in many African populations because of nutritional deficiencies, infections such as malaria and hookworm, and hemoglobinopathies. Two studies in Zaire show the impact of transfusions on the AIDS epidemic. Children with sickle cell anemia had a seven-fold increased likelihood of being seropositive compared with an age-matched control group (5.4 percent vs. 0.8 percent), and seropositivity correlated with the number of prior transfusions. A second study examined the relationship between malaria and HIV infection at Mama Yemo Hospital in Kinshasa. Fourteen percent of children there had a history of blood transfusions, and malaria was the indication for more than two-thirds of pediatric transfusions. Chloroquine-resistant falciparum malaria has recently spread to Zaire. The researchers identified 10 seropositive children with malaria who had received a transfusion during the current hospitalization, and four of these children were seronegative prior to transfusion. This study illustrates the complex epidemiology of AIDS by demonstrating how the resurgence of a tropical disease such as malaria, due in part to increasing chloroquine resistance, may accelerate HIV transmission through increased requirements for blood transfusions. The World Health Organization is helping to introduce HIV screening of blood donors in Africa.

Perinatal transmission

Although the female-to-male sex ratio for AIDS cases is 1:1, the ratio during peak child-bearing years is as high as 3:1 (Figure 1). The sex ratio for prevalence of serum antibody to HIV is similar. Because young women represent such a high proportion of HIV carriers, and because birth rates are so high in Africa, vertical transmission of HIV from infected mother to offspring is a major public health problem. Surveys of pregnant women have yielded HIV antibody prevalence rates of 2.6 percent in Nairobi, Kenya; 8 percent in Kinshasa, Zaire; 8.7 percent in Lusaka, Zambia; and 14 percent in Kampala, Uganda.

The risks of congenital, perinatal, and postnatal HIV transmission have not yet been clearly defined. A study in progress in two hospitals in Kinshasa, Zaire, suggests that the risk of congenital transmission may vary widely for different populations. The rate of virus isolation from cord blood of infants of seropositive women was 13/39 in the hospital serving the poor, and 2/26 in the hospital serving the more affluent. One factor that might account for this difference was the poorer general state of health and more advanced HIV-related disease in women from the former hospital. As appears to be the case with heterosexual transmission, this study found that transplacental infection of the fetus correlated with more pronounced immunosuppression (lower $T4/T8$ ratio) in the mother.

Although postnatal transmission, perhaps by breast feeding, has been well-documented in at least one case, its frequency is unknown. HIV can be isolated from breast milk, but it has yet to be shown that breast milk can be a vehicle for transmission. In the West, seropositive mothers are advised to forego breast feeding. In Africa, where bottle feeding is associated with appreciable infant morbidity and mortality due to diarrheal disease, HIV-related public health policies regarding breast feeding must await further information.

Discovery of HIV-2 in West Africa

During the past two years, a new human immunodeficiency virus termed HIV-2 has been discovered in West Africa. Although HIV-2 differs from HIV-1 over a substantial portion of its genome (see "Human Immunodeficiency Viruses and Related Simian AIDS Retroviruses" on page 16), it clearly can cause a syndrome identical to AIDS. It remains to be seen whether differences in the clinical features and epidemiology of HIV-1 and HIV-2 will eventually be defined. So far, the highest prevalence of HIV-2 has been found in prostitutes in West Africa, so it is probably sexually transmitted, as is HIV-1. The natural history and potential for further spread of HIV-2 remains to be defined. The differences in distribution of HIV-1 and HIV-2 in Africa are shown in Figure 2.

Impact on society

By 1991, it is predicted that 270,000 persons in the United States will have had AIDS. Costs for direct medical care in 1991 have been projected to be as high as $16 billion.

In the developing world, the economic impact will be comparatively greater. In African countries—where the per-capita annual health expenditure may be as low as $1 to $2—care of HIV-related illness may quickly drain all available health care resources. As many as 25 percent of adult and pediatric admissions in some Central African hospitals currently are HIV-related. The AIDS epidemic also may have an adverse impact on other diseases important in the Third World. For example, HIV-infected persons may have an attenuated response

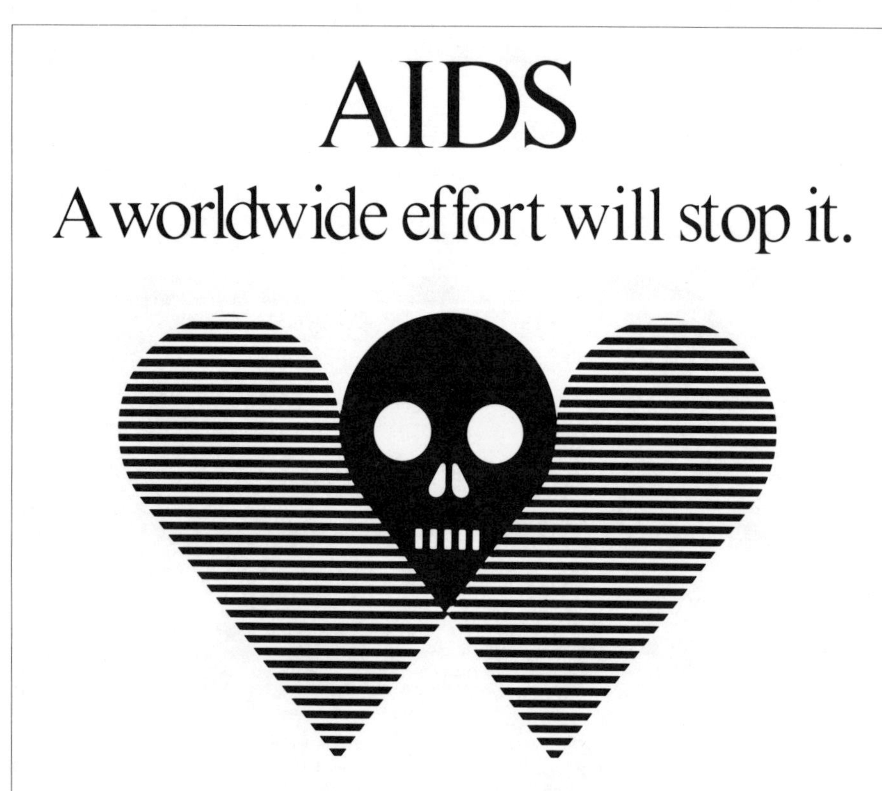

FIGURE 3. This logo is used worldwide in the AIDS control effort coordinated by the World Health Organization's Special Programme on AIDS.

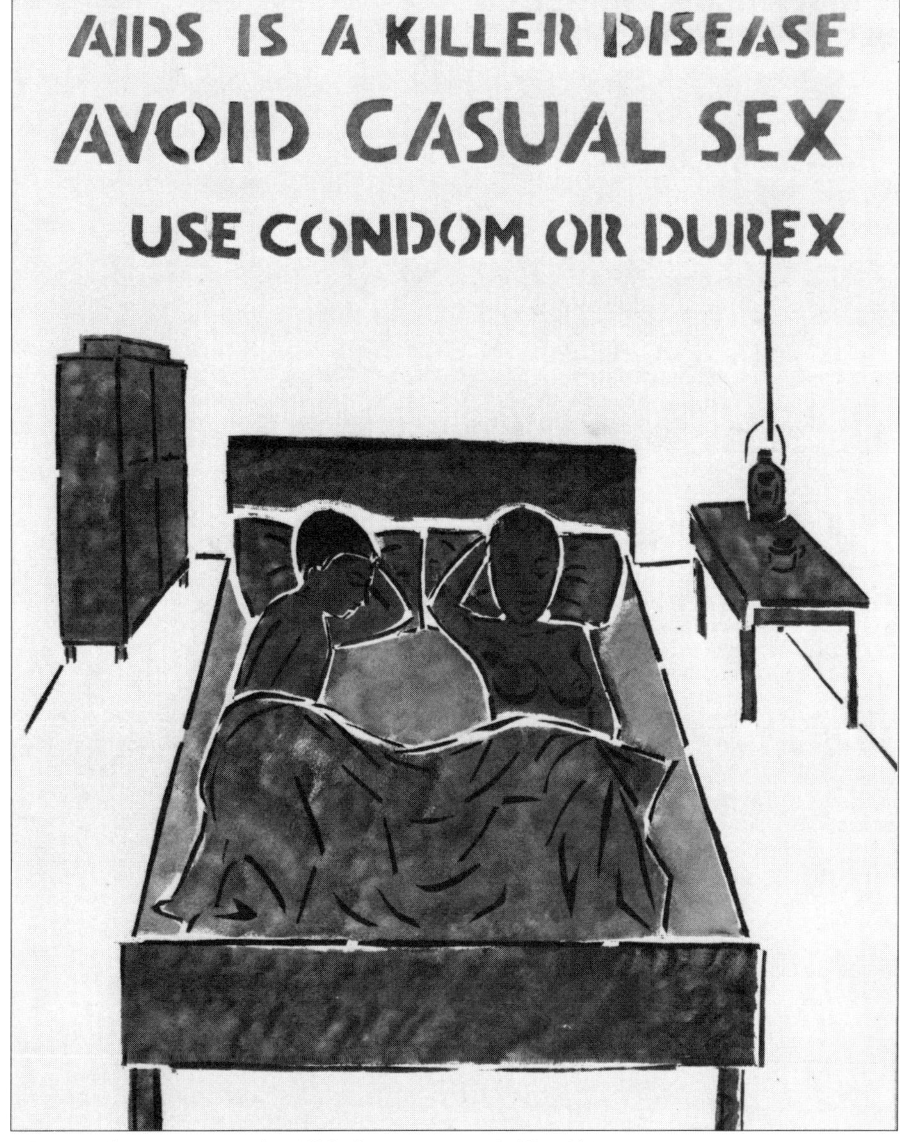

FIGURE 4. This poster is part of an AIDS education program in West Africa.

to vaccines. As the number of children with perinatal HIV infection grows, herd immunity to diseases such as measles or polio may be reduced sufficiently to allow epidemics to sweep through communities. Furthermore, the virulence of various diseases such as tuberculosis appears to be enhanced in persons with HIV infection. Thus, HIV may increase the transmissibility of tuberculosis and other communicable diseases. HIV infection is already thought to have slowed the decline in incidence of tuberculosis in the United States.

The economic impact of the AIDS epidemic can be measured not only in health care costs but also in the loss of years of productive life. Worldwide, persons in the 20-to-40 age range are at greatest risk for HIV infection. In some African countries, 20 percent or more of young urban adults—a considerable portion of the productive work force—have already been infected with HIV. Since women are a high percentage of infected young adults, perinatal transmission will result in substantial infant and childhood mortality in the next generation. Thus, HIV infection already has become firmly entrenched in some populations, both in the present generation and in the next.

Control of the epidemic

Global efforts to halt the spread of HIV infection are urgently needed. Government leaders, donor agencies, the scientific community and the general public have begun in the past year to appreciate the potentially catastrophic consequences of the AIDS epidemic. The African response illustrates this change in perception. As of June 1987, almost every African nation had requested assistance from the World Health Organization's Special Programme on AIDS (Figure 3). This is not yet true of many countries in Asia.

Without effective, inexpensive and widely available antiviral therapeutic options, the highest priority is to prevent transmission. With sexual transmission responsible for the majority of adult infections, public health education promoting condom use and discouraging multiple sexual partners will have the greatest impact (Figure 4). It is now well-documented that sexual prac-

tices among homosexual men in the United States and among some groups of prostitutes in Africa have changed dramatically in response to educational programs. The percentage of Nairobi prostitutes reporting some condom use rose from 8 percent in 1985 to more than 90 percent by 1987, due in part to an education campaign by the Kenyan Ministry of Health. HIV education programs need to be integrated with sexually transmitted disease control, family planning, and maternal and child health programs at local, state, national and international levels. Many countries are implementing two important strategies, blood-bank screening and sterilization of injection equipment, to reduce HIV transmission.

The potential for rapid spread of HIV within high-risk populations has been demonstrated in developing countries, as in developed countries. As mentioned above, in a cohort of African prostitutes negative for HIV serum antibody who were followed from 1985 to 1987, two-thirds developed HIV antibodies during that period. Perhaps even more alarming is the rate of spread within a low-risk population. In a study of hospital workers in Kinshasa, the incidence of HIV infection (seroconversion) from 1984 to 1985 was almost 1 percent. In the face of such an explosive and deadly pandemic, a coordinated international approach is required if control efforts are to be successful.

Additional Reading

AIDS—a public health crisis. Population Reports, Series L, number 6, July-August 1986.

Quinn, T.C., Mann, J.M., Curran, J.W., Piot, P. 1986. AIDS in Africa: an epidemiologic paradigm. *Science* 234:955-963.

Kreiss, J.K., Koech, D., Plummer, F.A. *et al.* 1986. AIDS virus infection in Nairobi prostitutes: spread of the epidemic to East Africa. *N Engl J Med* 314:414-418.

Van de Perre, P., Rouvroy, D., LePage, P. *et al.* 1984. Acquired immunodeficiency syndrome in Rwanda. *Lancet* ii:62-65.

Serwadda, D., Mugerwa, R.D., Sewankambo, N.K. *et al.* 1985. Slim disease: a new disease in Uganda and its association with HTLV-III infection. *Lancet* ii:849-852.

Mann, J.M., Francis, H., Quinn, T.C. *et al.* 1986. HIV seroprevalence among hospital workers in Kinshasa, Zaire. *JAMA* 256:3099-3102.

Piot, P., Plummer, F.A., Rey, M.A. *et al.* 1987. Retrospective seroepidemiology of AIDS virus infection in Nairobi populations. *J Inf Dis* 115:1108-1112.

A University of Washington Historical Connection: The Detection of HIV in Central Africa in 1959

by Arno G. Motulsky, M.D., Sc.D.
Editor, *University of Washington Medicine*

In 1957 I was asked to set up a unit of medical genetics in the Department of Medicine at the University of Washington. I worked out a rapid screening test for G6PD deficiency—a genetic trait particularly common in persons of African origin—and planned to test whether the trait's high frequency in tropical and subtropical countries was caused by a survival advantage of its carriers vis-a-vis falciparum malaria.

With the help of the Rockefeller Foundation, I made an extended field trip to Central Africa and to Sardinia in early 1959 to test this hypothesis. The test involved correlating the frequency of G6PD deficiency with malarial endemicity in various populations with high and low frequencies. I drew many blood specimens from malarial and non-malarial populations in the Belgian Congo (now Zaire), Rwanda and Burundi (then Belgian colonies). The malarial hypothesis ultimately turned out to be correct. Dr. Eloise Giblett, the recently retired director of the Puget Sound Blood Center, also tested the blood specimens for many other genetic traits. Leftover sera were kept in refrigerated storage.

After a test for AIDS was discovered in the 1980s, researchers began to test sera from various time periods in different parts of the world to learn the temporal and geographic origin of AIDS. Many specimens were tested, including the stored sera I had collected in Central Africa. Among nearly 700 sera from 1959, a single Congo specimen from Kinshasa (then Leopoldville) showed a positive result for the human im-

munodeficiency virus (HIV) with enzyme immunoassay testing and with confirmatory tests that included Western blot, immunofluorescence and immunoprecipitation (*Lancet* i:1279 - 1280, 1986). The specimen was obtained from a black, healthy, male subject who was both G6PD deficient and had the sickling trait. It was impossible to trace the young man from whom the specimen had been taken, since it was obtained anonymously from normals in Kinshasa. We know nothing, therefore, about his health status in the intervening years.

It was probably fortuitous that the man had both the sickling trait and G6PD deficiency, since 2 to 3 percent of the Kinshasa population carried both traits. However, no study has yet been done on the frequency of the sickling and G6PD deficiency traits among those infected with HIV.

This blood specimen is the earliest HIV-positive serum found so far and is the first documented case of an HIV infection. Its detection in Central Africa is consistent with other data that suggest a Central African origin of the HIV endemic that is sweeping the globe. It may be that HIV has been present in humans in Central Africa for long periods but has begun to spread more widely because of sociocultural changes such as urbanization, increased travel, and prostitution.

Dr. Motulsky is a University of Washington professor of medicine and genetics and is director of the Center for Inherited Diseases.

Glossary of Terms

This compilation includes commonly used acronyms and synonyms, components of various systems to clarify functional groups, and additional information for some terms that were not discussed in detail in the text.

AIDS: acquired immunodeficiency syndrome

ATEU: AIDS Treatment Evaluation Unit

ARC: AIDS-related complex

art/trs : anti-repression *trans*-activator/*trans*-regulator of splicing gene

AZT: azidothymidine, now known as zidovudine. The acronym AZT should no longer be used for this agent because, as of March 1987, it refers to a drug not related to AIDS treatment that is registered in another country. Zidovudine is the new generic name for azidothymidine.

CDC: Centers for Disease Control

ELISA: enzyme-linked immunosorbent assay

HIV: human immunodeficiency virus (two types). HIV-1 was known as HTLV-III, ARV and LAV-1; HIV-2 was known as LAV-2.

HIV antigens: translational protein products of the HIV gene ("p" is protein; "gp" is glycoprotein; number is molecular weight ratio in kilodaltons)

    p18
    p24
    gp41
    gp120
    gp160

HIV genes:
Accessory (regulatory) genes:

    sor
    *tat*III
    art/trs
    3'-*orf*

Structural HIV genes:

    gag
    pol
    env

HTLV-I, -II: human T-cell lymphotropic virus (two types)

IL-2 (interleukin-2): a glycoprotein lymphokine released by T-lymphocytes on stimulation with an antigen; functions as a T-cell growth factor by inducing proliferation of activated T-cells

LAV-1, -2: lymphadenopathy-associated virus (two types), now termed HIV-1 and HIV-2

LTR: long terminal repeat segment of HIV genome

MAI: *Mycobacterium avium-intracellulare*

orf : open reading frame

PCP: *Pneumocystis carinii* pneumonia

PHA: phytohemagglutinin; a protein with mitogenic activity that is derived from the red kidney bean

Provirus: A DNA copy of an animal retrovirus is integrated into the chromosome of the host cell, and thereby is present in all of the host's daughter cells.

Reverse transcriptase: retroviral enzyme that synthesizes DNA from RNA template

SAIDS-D virus: simian acquired immunodeficiency syndrome virus type D

SIV: simian immunodeficiency virus

sor : short open reading (frame)

***tat* III:** *trans*-activating transcriptional gene; see also HIV genes

T4 lymphocyte: also known as CD4 lymphocyte and as T helper/inducer lymphocyte

T4 receptor: also known as CD4 receptor

T8 lymphocyte: also known as CD8 lymphocyte and as T suppressor lymphocyte

T4/T8 (CD4/CD8) ratio: normal range is 1 or greater; AIDS range is less than 1.